CW00537777

THE
ART OF
ORAL
SEX

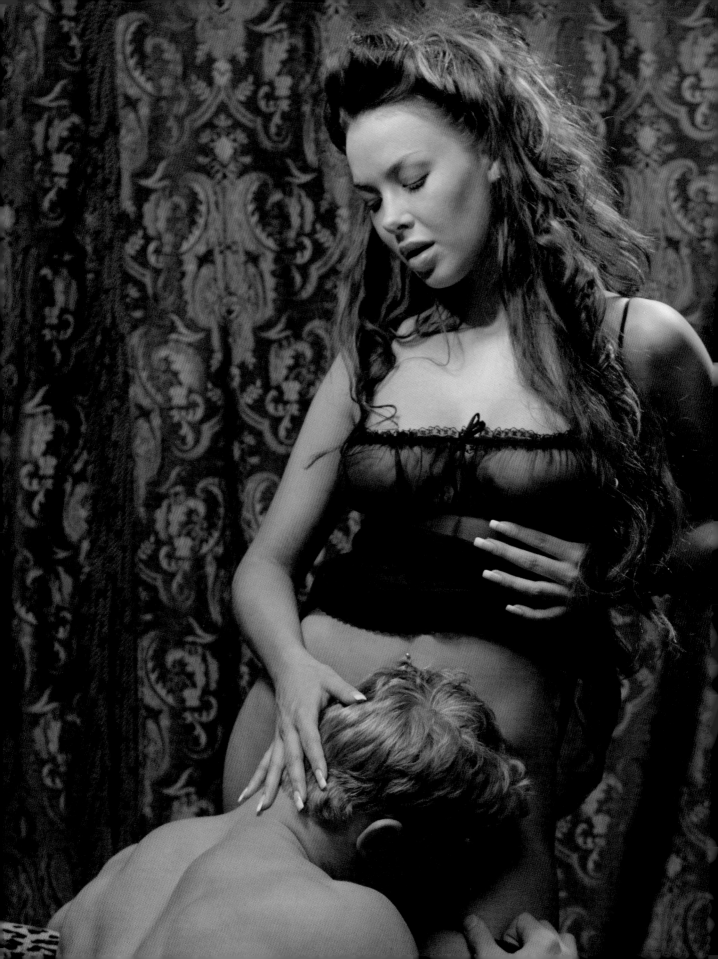

THE
ART OF
ORAL
SEX

BRING YOUR PARTNER TO NEW HEIGHTS OF PLEASURE

Advanced Techniques for Him and Her

Ian & Alicia Denchasy

QUIVER

Text and photography © 2007 by Quiver

First published in the USA in 2007 by
Quiver, a member of
Quayside Publishing Group
100 Cummings Center
Suite 406-L
Beverly, MA 01915-6101
www.quiverbooks.com

All rights reserved. No part of this book may be reproduced or utilized, in any form or by any means, electronic or mechanical, without prior permission in writing from the publisher.

The Publisher maintains the records relating to images in this book required by 18 USC 2257 which are located at Rockport Publishers, Inc., 100 Cummings Center, Suite 406-L, Beverly, MA 01915-6101.

11 10   5 6 7 8 9

ISBN-13: 978-1-59233-290-8
ISBN-10: 1-59233-290-0

Library of Congress Cataloging-in-Publication Data

Denchasy, Ian.
     The art of oral sex: bring your partnter to new heights of pleasure
using advanced techniques for him and her / Ian and Alicia Denchasy.
          p.   cm.
     ISBN 1-59233-290-0
     1. Oral sex.   I. Denchasy, Alicia. II. Title
HQ31.D427 2007
306.77'4--dc22

                                                                2007024409

Cover design and book design by Carol Holtz
Female model Sophia Santi, represented by Digital Playground

Printed and bound in Singapore

DEDICATION

*This book is dedicated to everyone who believes in
healthy marriages, strong relationships, and putting the needs
of others before their own.*

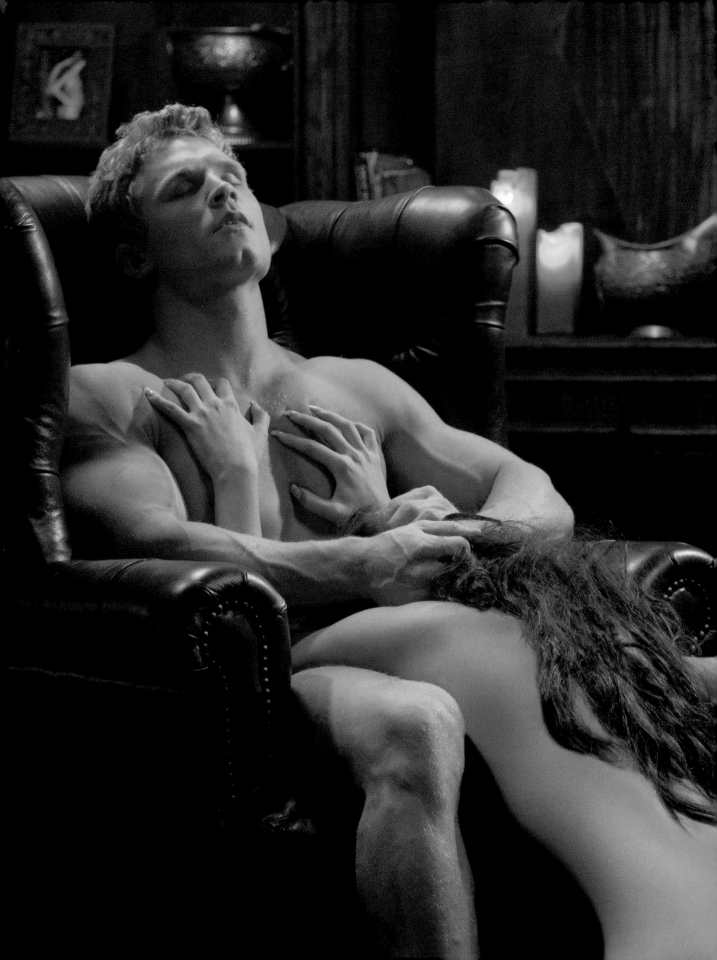

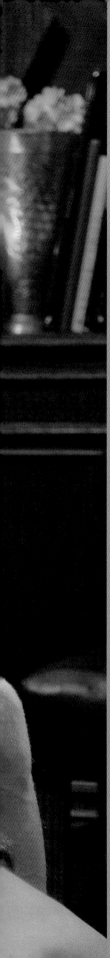

CONTENTS

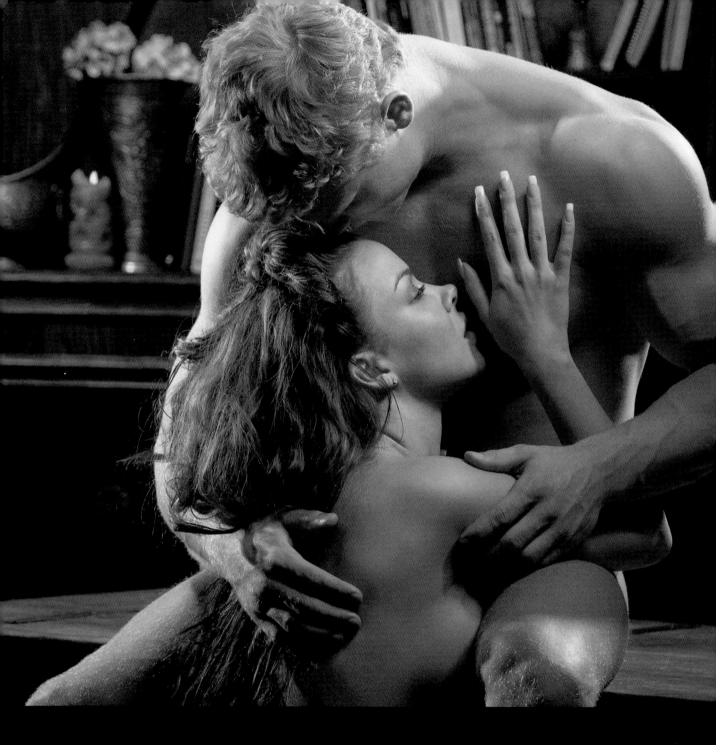

"*A man might forget* where he parks or where he lives, but he never forgets oral sex, no matter how bad it is."

—BARBARA BUSH
FORMER FIRST LADY OF THE UNITED STATES

INTRODUCTION

ON YOUR NEXT EXCURSION through the fabric of the World Wide Web, click over to Amazon and type "oral sex" in its search field. Then, do the same for the terms "cunnilingus" and "fellatio," respectively, and examine the results. As we write this introduction, our numbers are as follows: 9,156 search results for "oral sex," 2,048 for "cunnilingus," and more than 4,200 for "fellatio." By contrast, a mere 5,800 results are generated for "rocket science." It seems that there is a great deal to say about two of the most simple sexual acts known to human kind; or perhaps, the prospect of flying into outer space pales in comparison to giving good head or eating a tasty pussy.

So what's the big deal? Why is so much energy expended writing (and reading) about an act that seems, superficially, to be no more complex than eating a juice bar or biting into a ripe piece of fruit? Is oral sex *really* so difficult a subject that more words are assigned to its intricacies than sending human beings into space? And what, exactly, can a milquetoast couple living behind a white picket fence in a generic American neighborhood possibly add to a topic covered thousands of times before our entry into the fray? Indeed, we're wondering ourselves.

Hence, with respect to the thousands of oral sex experts who've come before us, we present this book as an *alternative* to the expected: an anti-oral sex book, if you will. Instead of simply focusing on blow jobs and pussy licking, we'll instead explore "going down" from the first tingle in our brains to the finality of orgasm and everything in-between. Certainly this treatise will include devotions to technique and form, but so much more will be discussed. In our investigations we'll touch on subjects including oral sex history, grooming, body and self image, hygiene, communication, desire, and couples-centric techniques to help us better become skilled artists in all things oral. And fabulous, hot photos will guide us along the way!

Whether it's proper grooming techniques, an anatomy lesson, or a treatise in maximizing orgasm from one of today's leading Tantra experts, we'll attempt to unravel the mysteries and enhance your knowledge of all things fellatio and cunnilingus and everything surrounding these sexual staples. And we'll do so—always—with both of you in mind.

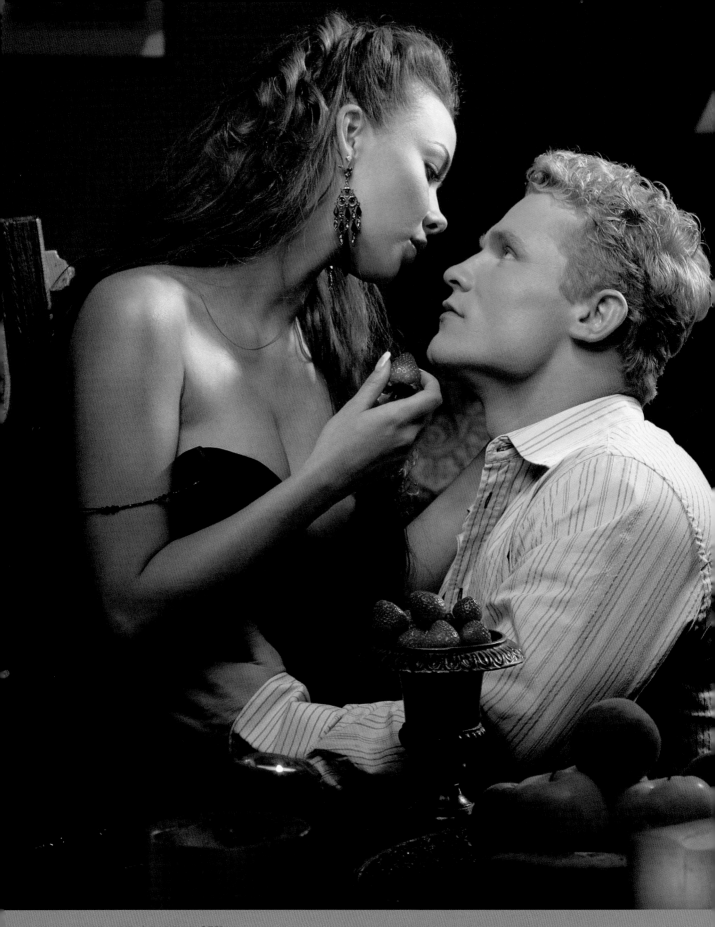

ABOUT THE AUTHORS

IN 2001, we unintentionally entered the "adult" world, leaving careers in teaching and law, respectively, in search of deeper sexual connection within the context of our then twelve-year marriage. Understanding that intimacy and love are vital to sustaining long-term relationships of any substance, we set about attempting to "spice up" what we considered a healthy sex life. Consulting adult websites for information, trying sex toys, watching adult videos, and visiting sex shops all over Los Angeles helped us discover ideas to achieve hotter days and steamier nights. Having literally zero experience in adult shopping or sexual research, we stumbled about blindly through stores, books, and websites without much success until, as luck would have it, we discovered a hidden treasure buried beneath a pile of socks in a dresser drawer.

That item, a vibrator called a Pocket Rocket, would prove to be a catalyst of sorts. Not only did it launch our sex life to new levels we'd never thought possible, but it inspired an entire life and career change as well. Besides leading us to true female orgasm for the first time, the Pocket Rocket motivated us to seek out additional toys and sexually stimulating items of all kinds, including (but certainly not limited to) flavored lubricants, penetration and multipurpose vibrators, dildos, anal stimulators, adult videos, erotic stories, cock rings, pheromones, massage oils, and even the occasional S&M item. Predictably, our sexual activity increased tremendously and has continued at its scorching pace ever since. (Indeed, we challenge couples twenty years our junior to keep up with our torrid rate!)

"*Take the attitude* of a student, never be too big to ask questions, never know too much to learn something new."

—OG MANDINO
AUTHOR OF *THE GREATEST SALESMAN IN THE WORLD*

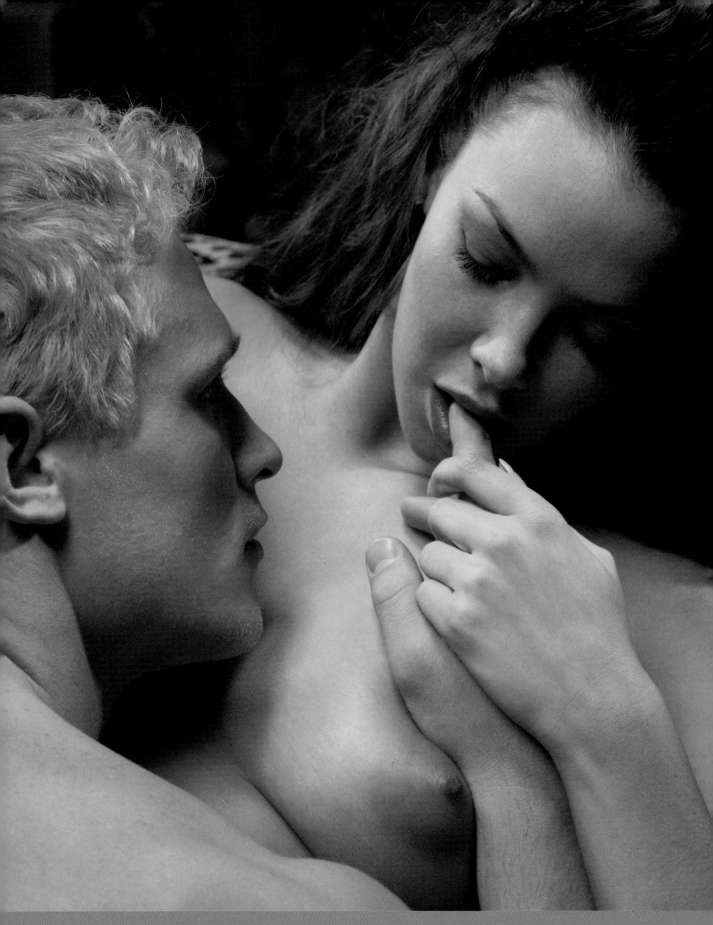

To finance our voracious appetite for all of these sexy new additions, we founded a website whose sole function would be to provide honest, impartial reviews of sexual enhancements within the context of committed relationships. In other words, we created an adult website for couples. Any toy, novelty, or other sexual product we acquired would be thoroughly reviewed and evaluated based upon its ability to provide pleasure to *both* of us. A clitoral vibrator, for example, is examined from the standpoint of whether or not it can be utilized easily while engaged in intercourse *and* in various positions. (A more traditional assessment would be based on self pleasure in isolation.)

It was our hope, with this endeavor, that manufacturers would send us anything and everything they had, thereby giving us never-ending reasons to keep on—for lack of a better term—*fucking and sucking* for the rest of our lives. Today, we can certainly say: "Mission accomplished!" Not only did manufacturers send boxes upon boxes of fun stuff to try, but our website grew exponentially over the years to become a viable business. We serve thousands of customers of all kinds who share our goals for strong relationships and healthy intimacy.

It is our sincere belief that intimacy plays a vital role in maintaining long-term relationships, and we therefore commit ourselves to providing tips and information consistent with that core principle. *The Art of Oral Sex* follows that tenet and is written to explore the marvels of oral sex as they pertain to you *both*, so we encourage you to enjoy this book together, open your hearts, unzip your imaginations, and plunge into the lower regions of sexual bliss.

The Art of Oral Sex is written to explore the marvels of oral sex as they pertain to you both, so we encourage you to enjoy this book together.

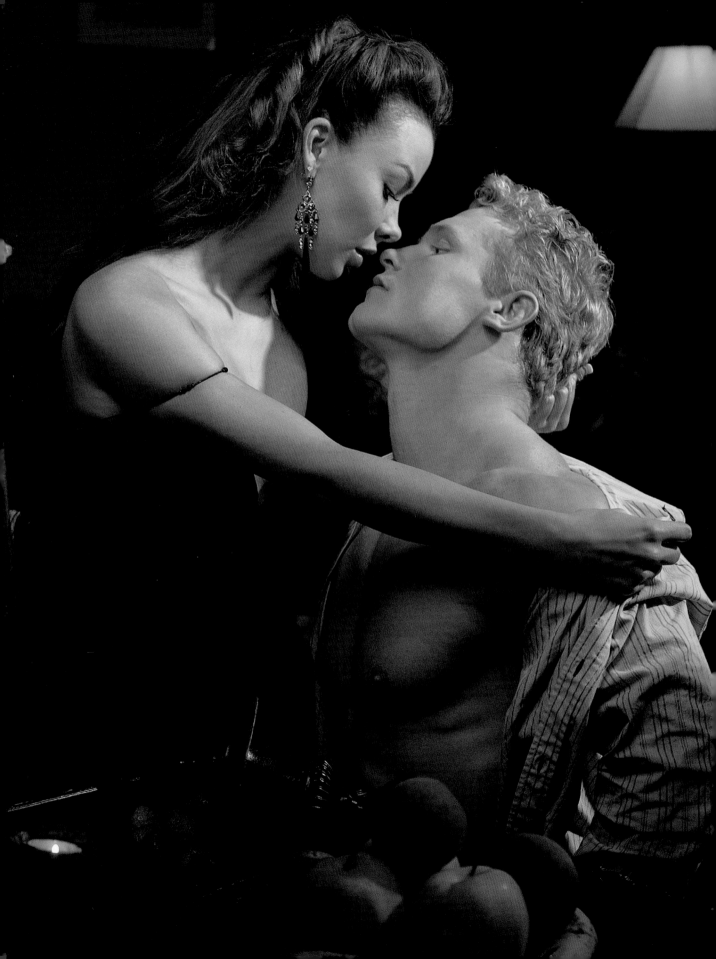

1

CHANNELING YOUR INNER ARTIST:

Know Your Subject

"One of the key ingredients in a good relationship is open, honest communication. First you have to feel safe, then you have to know what you want for yourself and how to say that, then you have to tell your lover how you think [and] feel, [and] what you need and want."

—DR. PATTI BRITTON
SEXOLOGIST AND AUTHOR OF
THE COMPLETE IDIOT'S GUIDE TO SENSUAL MASSAGE

TO CREATE A TRULY GREAT masterpiece, an artist must possess more than just extraordinary skill; indeed, Vincent van Gogh's *Irises* isn't one of the world's priceless treasures because it's a paint-by-number reproduction of something he saw while walking the grounds of Saint-Paul-de-Mausole. According to the artist himself, the work was an honest attempt to keep him from going insane. Such honesty and willingness to confront one's fears, joys, and intellectual curiosities is the hallmark of turning the mundane into the profound, and nowhere is this truth more evident than in the exploration of love and intimacy.

For us as couples to truly thrive and acheive lifetimes of happiness—to become great artists in our relationships to one another—we must first be willing to confront our deepest feelings, share them with our partners, and explore their implications together. Our sexuality, unfortunately, is likely the most difficult subject about which we can be honest; therefore, we are limited in our abilities to unlock its true potential. This blockage to true sexual openness can even result in dire consequences, such as separation and/or divorce—an end road no one wants to take (and certainly not if you're reading this book).

EMBRACING THE ART OF ORAL SEX

Oral sex, or "going down" brings with it an entirely unique set of challenges and rewards. It is an activity that falls under the term "sodomy," which is defined as "sexual acts that are not intended for the purpose of procreation." The fact remains that there are still laws throughout the world in which a person caught in the act of oral sex can be prosecuted, jailed, and, in rare cases, put to death. (Even in the United States, up until 1950, every state had laws banning nonprocreative sex.)

Considering the relatively recent acceptance of nonprocreative sex and freedom from persecution, it's no wonder so many books, videos, and lectures are produced yearly on the subjects of cunnilingus and fellatio. Indeed, it will probably take a few more generations to fully purge ourselves of the residual guilt handed down by our forefathers against such heavenly acts of love.

History aside, many—if not most—modern couples enjoy some form of oral pleasure, if only a kiss or mild lick or two. Going down provides a wonderful warm-up to sexual intercourse, assisting with both mental and physical lubrication. It paves the way for increased intensity of orgasm and instills a deeper appreciation for the beauty of our reproductive organs. Enjoyed on its own, going down can elicit explosive sexual encounters every bit as passionate as intercourse. In fact, with a few skillful moves, your lover may request your hands and mouth more often than you think!

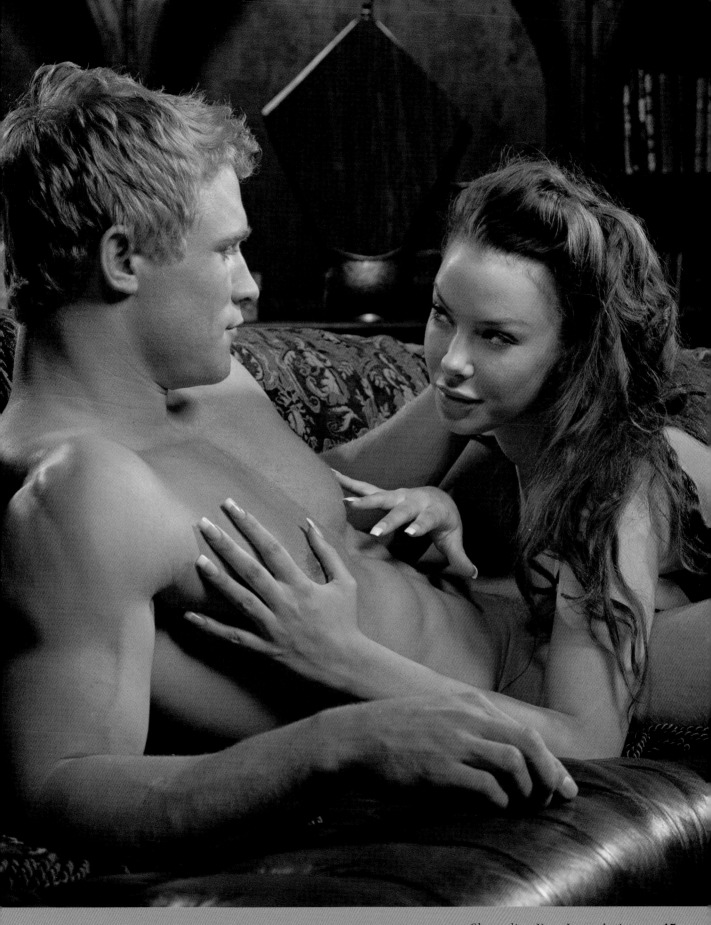

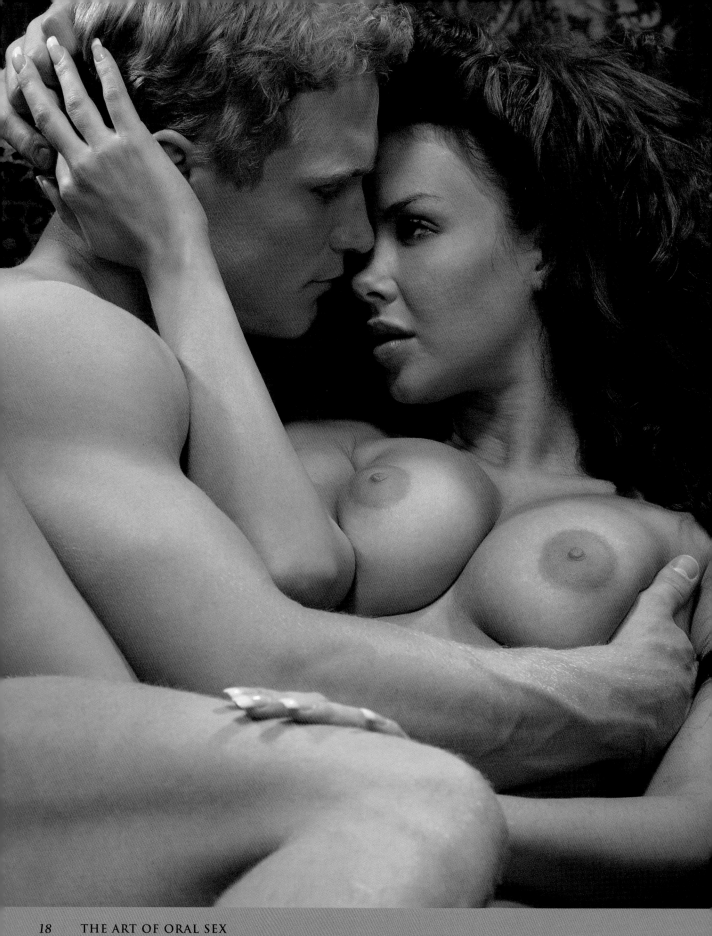

TALKING ABOUT GOING DOWN

To completely fulfill an exciting adventure down under, it's vital that you understand and communicate exactly what adventure you want. For many of us—whether together forty days or forty years—expressing our sexual desires is uncomfortable and awkward. With religious, cultural, and societal pressures telling us what's acceptable, we are often conflicted and confused as to what we *really* want in our sexual relationships. Add to that the uncertainty of how your partner will react to your desires and it's understandable that you might be hesitant to share your deepest cravings. No one wants to face the prospect of a shocked or turned-off partner thinking: "You want me to do *what?!*"

In our marriage, for example, we both sulked for weeks when our sexual activity dropped following the birth of our son; however, a simple (yet deep) conversation eventually led to some minor life adjustments, putting us back on track. Wouldn't it have been better to lay our cards on the table immediately, rather than endure weeks of cold shoulders and shallow, icy conversations?

TANTALIZING TIPS

❧ Cunnilingus is a great opportunity to practice sexual communication skills. Tell your partner you will do *only* as she directs, letting her control every aspect of your dining experience. If she is hesitant, simply stay patient and kiss the area lightly, reassuringly asking for guidance. With a little practice, she'll take charge of her orgasm and you'll both be treated with intense and meaningful results. The same technique can be used with fellatio.

❧ Once every other week, send your lover an email describing one sexual or sensual act that you either love or want to try. Invite your lover to do the same on alternate weeks. It can be something you already do together ("I love it when you give me kisses all over my body") or something you've never requested or done before ("I'd love you to take my head in your lap and stroke my hair"). Fulfill your respective requests the following Saturday night, or on any mutually-agreed-upon evening when you are free to pay attention to each other.

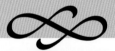

"*Have you heard* of this new book, 1001 Sexual Secrets Men Should Know? It contains comments from 1001 women on how men can be better in bed. I think that women would actually settle for three: slow down, turn off the TV, and call out the right name."

—JAY LENO
LATE NIGHT TALK SHOW HOST

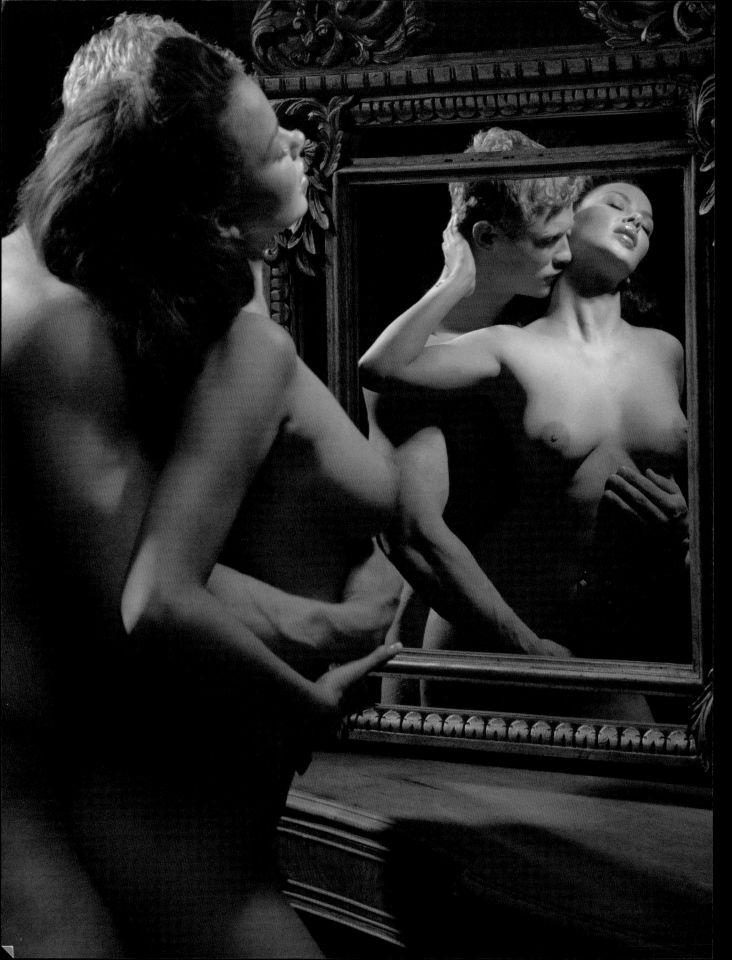

2

PREPARING YOUR CANVAS:

Readiness and Grooming

"I believe that what it is I have been called to do will make itself known when I have made myself ready."

—JAN PHILLIPS
AUTHOR OF *THE ART OF ORIGINAL THINKING*

WHEN ENGAGED IN ANY ART, whether it's sculpture, painting, drawing, or sexual frivolity, preparation is always the key to creating lasting impressions. Think of our bodies as beautiful canvasses upon which art shall be created. Every inch of our physical person should be primed and each of the five senses engaged; sight, which includes grooming and physical health; taste, which can include luscious flavors in the form of ointments, creams, and edibles; smells, which comprise fragrance, lotions, potions, and natural scents; touch, in which the bonding of human skin is heightened through increased circulation and texture; and finally sound, whereby the breath, voice, and auditory senses are aroused to heighten sexual awareness and enjoyment. Ideally, when all five senses are engaged, the chances of reaching the perfect orgasm are practically guaranteed.

THE ART OF GROOMING

In the HBO comedy series, *Curb Your Enthusiasm*, Larry David sits up in bed, his wife Cheryl purring from his implied oral skills, and he begins congratulating himself on his cunnilingus acumen. Suddenly, however, Larry begins gagging, blurting out, "I think I have a pubic hair in my throat!" This begins a long-running joke through the next three episodes, culminating with the expulsion of said pubic annoyance during a brawl in a nativity scene outside his Bel Air mansion. We kid you not. And while most sexual situations rarely rise to the comedic heights of Larry and Cheryl David, who among us has not experienced the perils of dislodged body hairs?

In the realm of the visual, our bodies are like canvases to which love is applied in fine brush strokes. Hence, preparing our bodies for receiving such attention begins with proper grooming. In other words, we should always try to look—and feel— our sexy best. From a simple trim to the meticulous permanent removal of hair, care should be taken to

DID YOU KNOW?

Pubic hair has practically no function biologically. Surprisingly, scientists have no definitive answer to why we have pubes, although they think pubic hair was once a mechanism for producing pheromones to help attract suitable mates. However, in modern societies we now cover our genital areas, rendering our mojos obsolete.

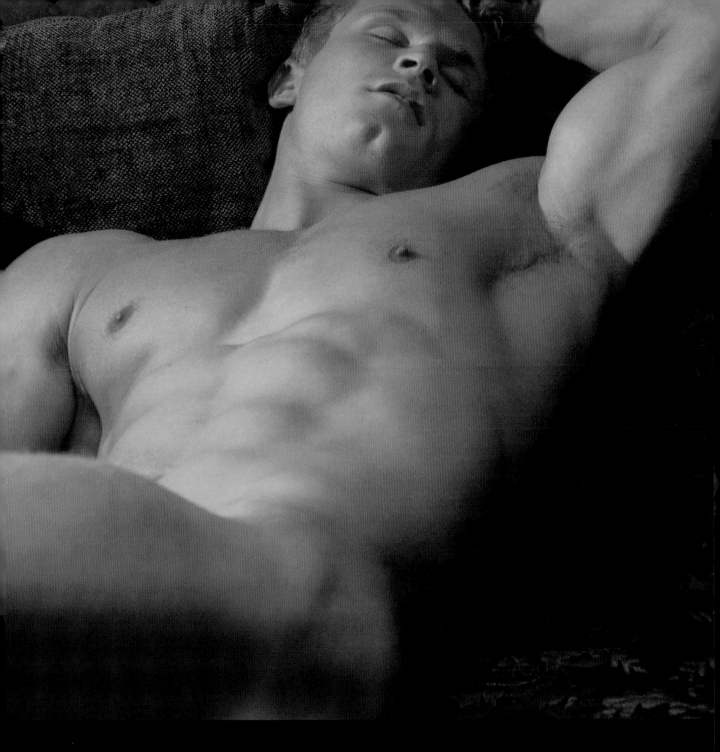

"Winning is like shaving—*you do it every day or you wind up looking like a bum.*"

—JACK KEMP

POLITICIAN AND FORMER PROFESSIONAL
AMERICAN FOOTBALL PLAYER

prepare our erogenous zones for maximum sensitivity and minimum interference. The male nipple area, for example, can provide a wonderful destination for his lover's tongue and fingers, especially without an overabundance of hair to block such exploration.

Navigating through thick jungle foliage to reach the mythical gold mines of El Dorado certainly would have been easier had the Spanish conquistadors had access to modern John Deere back hoes and Black and Decker chain saws—and so too should your best efforts be applied to the journey toward the sweetness of your lover's treasures. With these goals in mind, the most effective grooming methods available are outlined here. They all have their merits; choose the one that is right for you.

PERFORMANCE ART: *SHAVING PROPERLY*

There are several ways to clear the way for oral exploration, from expensive laser surgeries to hair removal creams and all manner of electronic devices designed to chop, smooth, and prepare the privates for pleasure. For value and closeness, however, very few methods can match the good, old-fashioned razor to get the job done right. With the right blend of patience, technique, and tools, you'll have it down to an erotic and pleasurable science in no time.

DID YOU KNOW?

In 2003, the U.S. Supreme Court handed down the *Lawrence et al.* v. *Texas* decision, which effectively overrides most state laws against sodomy, making non-procreative sex acts free from categorization as a crime.

- For males, start with the chest and back area, removing the majority of the hair with small scissors or an electric trimmer, both of which can be easily found at your local department store for around ten U.S. dollars. For females, do the same for the pubic region, paying close attention to the area around the labia and clitoris.

- Immediately following this initial stage, take a warm shower or bath to soften the hair, perhaps applying oil to the areas to be shaved to decrease irritation. Olive or grape seed oil work great.

- Pretreat the areas to be shaved with a simple hair conditioner. Most conditioners contain lanolin (a waxy substance derived from sheep's wool), which helps prevent razor burn by coating the skin with a protective layer, helping the razor glide more smoothly. If you're tempted to purchase expensive creams sold in adult stores or online, you needn't bother as they have little to no advantage over a ninety-nine-cent bottle of hair conditioner.

- Take your shaving cream or gel and lather up, the thicker the foam the better.

- Consider using a mirror—full length if you have one—to get a better view of things. Sit on a towel in a chair directly in front of it.

- Begin shaving from the top down, trying to confine your strokes to the direction of hair growth (if you can figure it out). Try to keep the number of strokes to a minimum and rinse the razor often in warm water.

- If shaving the testicles, make sure to pull the skin as flat as possible with your hand. Use downward strokes, gently grazing the hair with short, fluid movements. To get behind the testicles, grab and cradle them in the fingers of your opposite hand, then stroke from back to front. Make sure to shave the area between the anus and scrotum, rinsing the razor often to get more hair with each stroke.

- Rinse and gently pat the area dry.

- Finish by applying a hypoallergenic lotion, such as AHAVA or Jergens. Do *not* use any applications containing alcohol, such as aftershave, which can be very painful.

- If you get razor rash (trust us: you'll know it when you see it), treat the area with Neosporin ointment, almond oil, aloe, or cocoa butter until it subsides.

- Since you are almost guaranteed to itch when the hair begins to grow back, it might be a good idea to apply hypoallergenic lotion to help alleviate the discomfort.

- Immediately show your new creation to your lover and repeat as needed!

TANTALIZING TIPS

- Forget about plastic surgery and penis extensions! Did you know shaving off that big hairy mojo can actually make your penis look almost a third larger?

- Guys, don't forget to shave your face! Would you want sandpaper applied to your penis? If not, shave your face to avoid irritating her inner thighs and everything in-between.

- *Neat*, *Nair*, and *Magic Shave* are NOT for intimate shaving! You might be tempted to use hair removal products that promise to simply whisk away the hair after applying, but don't do it! Ingredients contained in these concoctions can irritate the vagina and are not effective against the coarse hair found in the pubic areas.

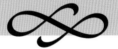

In the realm of the visual, our bodies are like canvases to which love is applied in fine brush strokes. Hence, preparing our bodies for receiving such attention begins with proper grooming.

INDUSTRIAL DESIGN:
POWERED SHAVERS AND GROOMING KITS

If placing a sharp object near your most intimate areas sounds a tad unappealing, you might wish to try one of the many products available to automate the process without the risk of errant blades. Typically, intimate shavers work in much the same way as electric razors for men's faces and women's legs, which separate the blades from direct epidermal contact via a thin metal "foil," dotted with tiny openings that allow hair to enter and be cut without irritation or damage to underlying skin. Unfortunately, pubic hair is often coarser than facial and body hair, especially in certain nationalities, meaning results can be disappointing for certain people. (Asian hair, for example, tends to fall into this category.) If you have an extra fifty to seventy-five U.S. dollars lying around, however, you might want to give one of these devices a try. Most of the powered personal shavers are manufactured by Seiko and Panasonic, with a smattering of others (Braun, Philips, Sanyo, Epilady, ConAir, and Sunbeam) making up the rest of the market. Oftentimes to sweeten the deal, the shavers will come as a kit, with one or two extra trimmers to remove the bulk of the hair prior to using the main unit. Whichever model you choose, however, here are some simple tips to help you get the most from your powered shaver:

- Using a trimmer or small pair of scissors, remove as much hair as possible.

- Take a warm bath or shower to soften the hair and open the pores.

- After towel drying, apply talc to desired shaving areas to thoroughly dry them before using the shaving unit. Dryness is key.

- Begin shaving, using small circular motions and pressing gently to remove all remaining hair.

- For best results, shave in front of a full length mirror, sitting in a chair to assist in seeing below the waist and preventing neck cramps.

- Make sure to empty the shaver foil frequently, as the buildup of talc and hair can slow the blades, resulting in less than optimum results.

- Plan to trim every two to three days, as the task is much easier when hair is short.

TANTALIZING TIP

Men, don't forget that trusty Norelco! If you already own an electric shaver, you may have everything you need for a close, smooth shave. Use the trimmer to whack away the majority of the hair, then simply shave the genital area as you would your face. Avoid the testicles, however, as an accidental "owie" might turn you into an opera singer.

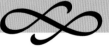

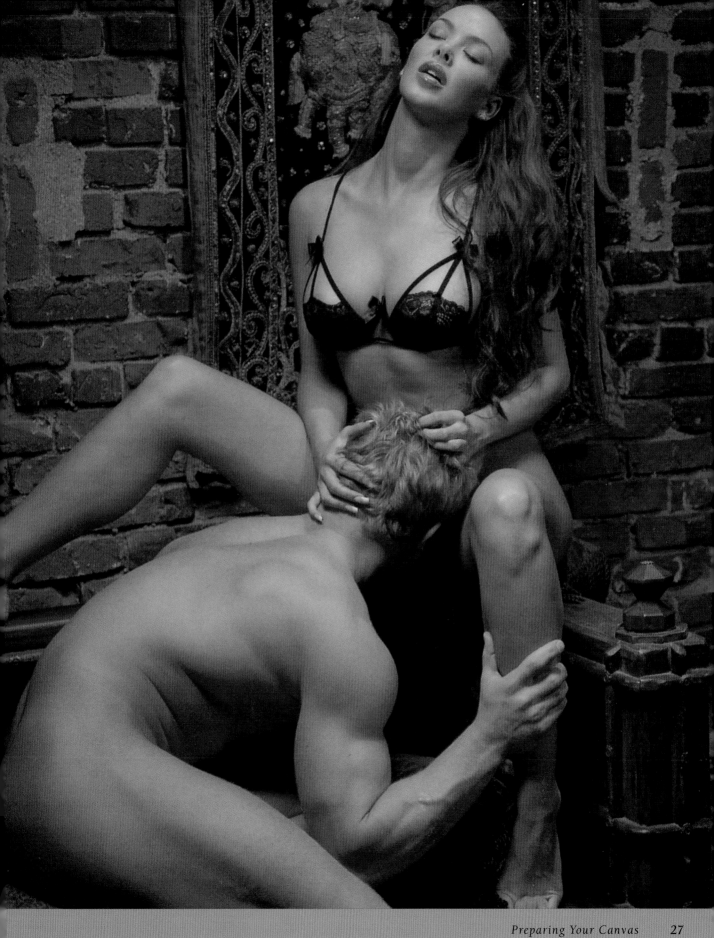

SCULPTURE: *WAXING AT HOME OR AT THE SALON*

If the thought of razors near your privates or the hassle of constant self-maintenance isn't your cup of tea, it may be time to visit your local spa or favorite salon for a waxing. In addition to getting the absolute closest hair removal of any method short of permanent solutions (like laser treatments), the skin is left smooth and soft for many days after each treatment. Furthermore, the more you wax, the softer the hair becomes and the less discomfort you will experience.

Speaking of pain, you will not be sent into stratospheric heights of profanity as your hair is ripped from its follicles—à la Steve Carell in *The Forty-Year-Old Virgin.* Yes, the first time hurts, sometimes a lot, but it subsides quickly if waxing is performed by licensed cosmetologists who know what they're doing. Besides, whatever happened to the "no pain, no gain" mantra? If you're at all apprehensive, YouTube is filled with videos showing facial expressions at the moment the wax is ripped from the skin, so you can judge for yourself if you're up to the challenge.

There are two types of waxing procedures most commonly performed: the standard bikini wax and the Brazilian. The former is mainly done on the

TANTALIZING TIP

Pubic hair can even be waxed and shaped into surprising and sexy patterns. Hearts are a popular option, but use your imagination. Dying the hair a new color is another bold move that might delight your lover.

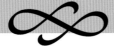

DID YOU KNOW?

If the thought of ripping out your genital hair seems too painful, you might want to talk to your doctor about getting a prescription for a topical pain reducing cream. Those containing lidocaine, tetracaine, menthol, and camphor can help ease the sting if applied before and/or after the waxing procedure.

areas where hair can be seen outside a typical bikini or bathing suit, while the latter is a more complex method that removes virtually all hair around the pubic area and anus, leaving only a small "landing strip" visible above the vulva.

Waxing begins with baby or talcum powder (or in some cases, oil) spread over the target area to be waxed, in order to prevent hot wax from adhering to the skin. The hot wax is then spread over the area, allowed to harden, then literally pulled (some would say "torn") off, taking the hair and upper dead skin cells with it. The procedure is then repeated over the rest of the desired areas (anus, butt, genital areas, chest, etc.) until the area is soft and smooth. Finally, any hairs not removed in the waxing procedure are removed with tweezers. If a "landing strip" or other shape is desired, scissors are used to trim it to finish.

Before you schedule your appointment, here are some additional facts worth knowing:

❦ Because pubic hair is thicker and coarser than most other body hair, different waxes should be used to remove it. Most often, this is a mixture of

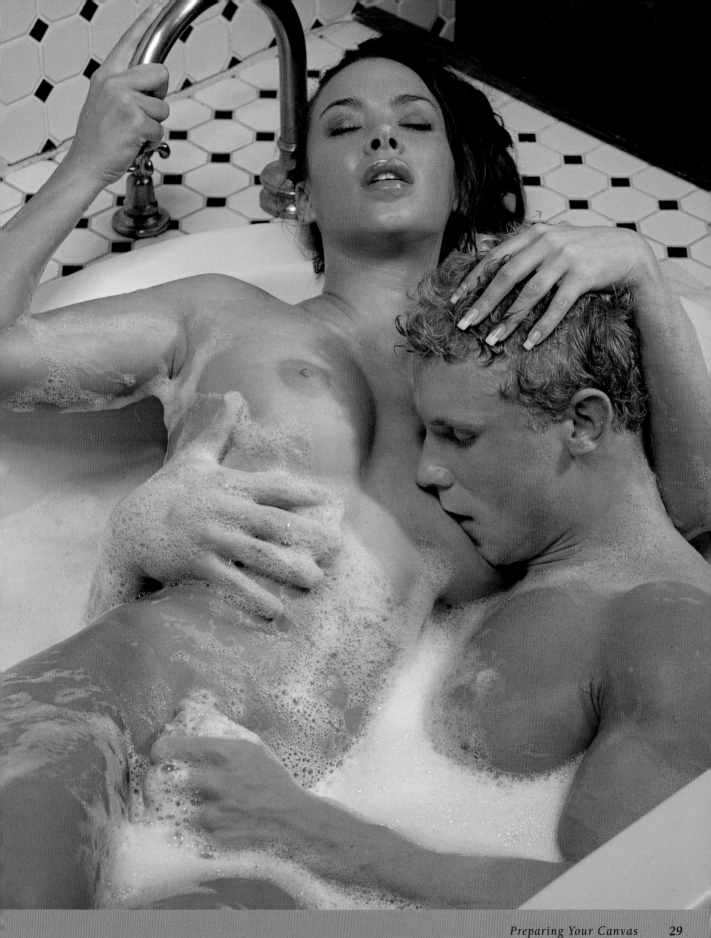

natural beeswax and oil, as this combination is stronger and more effective for pubic areas than synthetic waxes (which are used most commonly used to remove leg hair).

- Expect some pain. Depending on the esthetician's skill level performing the procedure, your own tolerance for pain, and your mental state going in, waxing may hurt a lot or a little. While the first time may cause mild to severe pain, many claim the pain lessens over time as you "get used to it." There are also topical anesthetics to help lessen the pain and most salons carry them just in case.

- Hair inhibitors, which slow hair regrowth, may be available at your waxing salon. These inhibitors cut down on visits (and save you money), so be sure to ask your salon about them.

- The benefits of pubic waxing are similar to those of other types of body waxing: lack of razor burn and soft hair regrowth. Compared to nonpubic body waxing, however, the disadvantage—pain—may be more acute (since the waxing is performed on an extremely sensitive region of the body).

There are now many home kits available to do the waxing yourself, but you will usually get better results with a licensed esthetician. Do your homework if you are at all unsure about the person performing your waxing (don't be afraid to ask to see their credentials if they aren't in plain sight).

THE PERMANENTLY BLANK CANVAS: *ELECTROLYSIS AND LASER TREATMENTS*

If the effort to maintain your "mojo" isn't for you, you might consider partial or full permanent removal of hair around your intimate areas. Though expensive, science has evolved quite dramatically in this area, now offering solutions using electrolysis or lasers to either prevent the follicles from growing hair completely, or inhibiting growth to the extent that the hair is barely visible to the naked eye. Beware, however, that even the best claims are just that—claims. The fact is that these solutions can sometimes be painful and anything but permanent. We recommend doing as much research as possible before engaging in any form of body alteration, be it hair removal or something more involved. Here's an overview of the two most common "permanent" hair removal solutions.

ELECTROLYSIS

Electrolysis is the practice of electrical epilation to permanently remove human hair. An electrologist is sometimes referred to as an "electrolysist" and the actual process of removing the hair is referred to as electrolysis. The practitioner slides a hair-thin

TANTALIZING TIP

Use grooming time as foreplay. Invite your partner to share a hair-softening bath or to apply your soothing lotion afterward. Done with the right attitude, even shaving can be sexy; the mind will be running with delicious thoughts of what is to come!

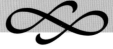

metal probe into each hair follicle. Proper insertion does not puncture the skin. Electricity is delivered to the follicle through the probe, which causes localized damage to the areas that generate hairs. Done properly, this effectively "kills" the follicle and theoretically no hair can ever regrow. Professional electrolysis is very expensive, and is usually charged by the hour; ten to twenty hours are required to fully treat a bikini area. Beware that this treatment method can be extremely painful and that many states unfortunately do not require any sort of certification for electrolysists. Proceed with extreme caution.

LASER TREATMENTS

Laser hair treatments are similar in cost to electrolysis, but laser hair removal works by sending a beam of laser light to a group of hair follicles with enough power to disable or destroy the root, but not enough power to harm the surrounding skin. This process is called "selective photothermolysis." It is selective because it targets only the hair and not the skin. Photo means "light" and thermolysis means "destroying with heat." The surrounding skin is usually cooled. Some methods include a gel, a spray, or a cooling tip.

The laser beam finds the hair follicles by targeting melanin, which is the substance that gives skin and hair dark color. Therefore, the ideal candidate for laser has dark hair and light skin. The laser will not work on people with red, white, gray, or true blond hair. The hot laser light will also be attracted to the melanin in the skin, so people with suntans, or dark skin types are at more of a risk for discoloration of pigment and other side effects.

DID YOU KNOW?

It may surprise you to know that the vagina is one of the *cleanest* parts of the human body, constantly cycling fluids through it to kill bacteria and keep its PH balance at optimum levels. Using too much soap or bathing too frequently actually has the opposite effect and can alter the PH levels and cause unpleasant odors.

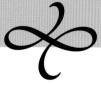

Laser only destroys hair in its active growth phase, the anagen phase. This phase lasts several years, and up to eighty-five percent of our hair is in that phase at any given time. The good thing is that during this phase, the hair has an abundance of melanin and the hair follicle is easily targeted.

THE RAZOR'S IN YOUR COURT

Whatever grooming method you choose, it is important to talk frankly to your partner about the results that make you both happy. If too much chest or back hair is preventing your tongue from reaching his nipples, don't be afraid to let him know! Are you a fan of big beautiful muffs? Tell her to put that razor down immediately. A little attention to your personal canvases can boost your own sexual perception and self image, transferring this positive energy toward being a more open and willing partner. It might even save you from a *Curb Your Enthusiasm* moment.

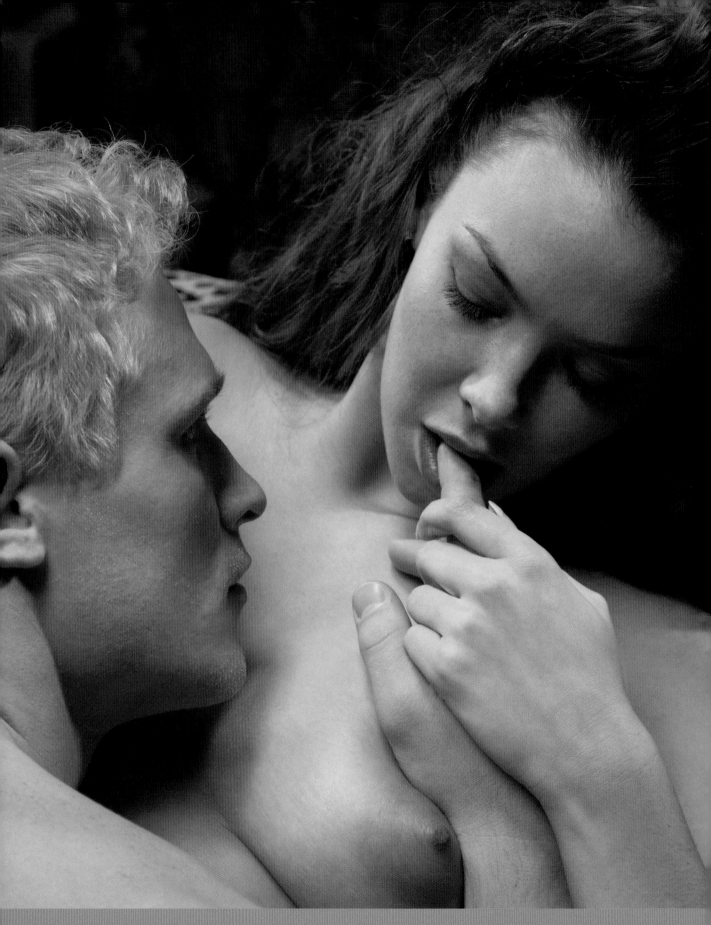

TASTES AND AROMAS OF LOVEMAKING

The taste of your lover should be savored, like a fine wine, so slow down and enjoy every mouth-watering flavor. In some cases, the taste of a woman can vary from the clitoris to the inner lips. When going down, the tongue is not only a source of pleasure for your partner, but, with your taste buds' sensitivity heightened, it can be a source of great pleasure to you as well.

Occasionally, however, we encounter a lover whose tastes are less than sweet. Why does this sometimes happen? Well, believe it or not, the foods we consume affect the taste of the substances we expel from our love nests. For the male, garlic, asparagus, coffee, and even meat can drastically affect the taste of his semen as these food increase acidity. Smoking can also cause bitterness, so it might be wise to avoid swishing his cum in your mouth the first few go rounds.

In females, her flavor and aroma can be affected by a multitude of factors, such as monthly cycles, stress, diet, and vitamins, and her natural juices can taste slightly sweet, salty, or even tangy. As with males, women should consume strong foods (such as asparagus, garlic, and artichokes) modestly. Both of you should get in the habit of drinking plenty of fluids to keep your sexual facilities in top condition.

DID YOU KNOW?

Sugars can change a woman's PH balance and cause yeast infections. Avoid applying substances containing sugar to the vaginal area.

"'Where should one use perfume?,' a young woman asked. 'Wherever one wants to be kissed,' I said."

—COCO CHANEL
FASHION DESIGNER

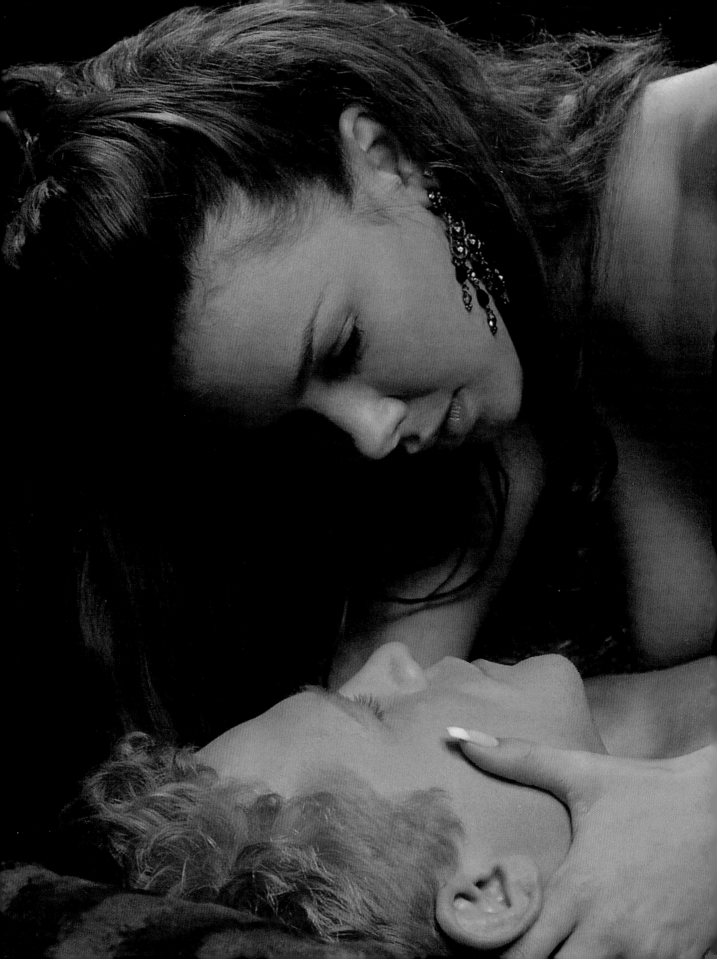

3

ASSEMBLE YOUR MATERIALS:

Sensual Anatomy 101

*"Anyone who believes that the way
to a man's heart is through his
stomach flunked geography."*

—ROBERT BYRNE
BILLIARDS CHAMPION AND NOVELIST

THE HUMAN FORM

To nourish your inner artist, no more important factor comes into play than *knowledge*. And when charting a course for love and intimacy, knowledge about your partner's "geography" is certainly key. The awareness of *where* your lover's pleasure points reside will determine, more than anything else, *how* you will conduct yourself in your duty to stimulate those areas. With your lips and hands as your tools, you must understand that oral gratification stretches well beyond the genital area, with millions of skin cells teeming with nerve receptors awaiting motivation. Indeed, the typical human body contains millions of nerve receptors located in the upper and lower layers of skin, capable of responding to pressure and temperature, sending signals directly to our brains. This ingenious mechanism of human evolution is so sensitive that, if blindfolded, we can feel another person's presence in the same room simply by the movement of air caused by his or her slight movements. It's no wonder blindfolds are so popular in sexual situations! When deprived of sight (our number one sense) our tactile senses are heightened to the point where we can "see" with our fingertips.

THE HEAD AND NECK

Though the region above the shoulders may seem obvious territory for erotic sensations, few lovers address this important area for more than a kiss on the lips or peck on the neck as they make their way downward. Ignoring the many opportunities for stimulation, however, can do both the giver and receiver of oral pleasure an enormous disservice. If you were a painter, would you simply paint the lips and neck, oblivious to the ears, chin, nose, eyes, forehead, and scalp? Would Jan Vermeer's *Girl with the Pearl Earring* or DaVinci's *Mona Lisa* capture the imaginations of millions were it not for the whole of their transfixing features?

The face is a wondrous abundance of opportunity for touching, caressing, licking, and exploring. Starting with a few strokes though your lover's hair, use your fingertips to gently massage the temples and closed eyelids, moving slowly around the ears and cheekbones, finally making your way down past the lips and under the chin, smoothly sweeping the muscles from the throat forward. Repeat the same motions with your lips and watch the goose bumps rise.

TANTALIZING TIP

Do not *blow* in your lover's ear; instead, move in close and simply breathe naturally for the best result. Also, now would be a great opportunity to whisper sweet "somethings" into his or her ear. Express how turned on you are and how lucky you feel to be the one giving him or her pleasure. Don't be afraid to throw a bit of naughtiness into your messages, either: letting him know how hungry you are for his cock, or conversely for her delicious pussy, can set things in motion for an explosive climax later.

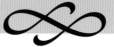

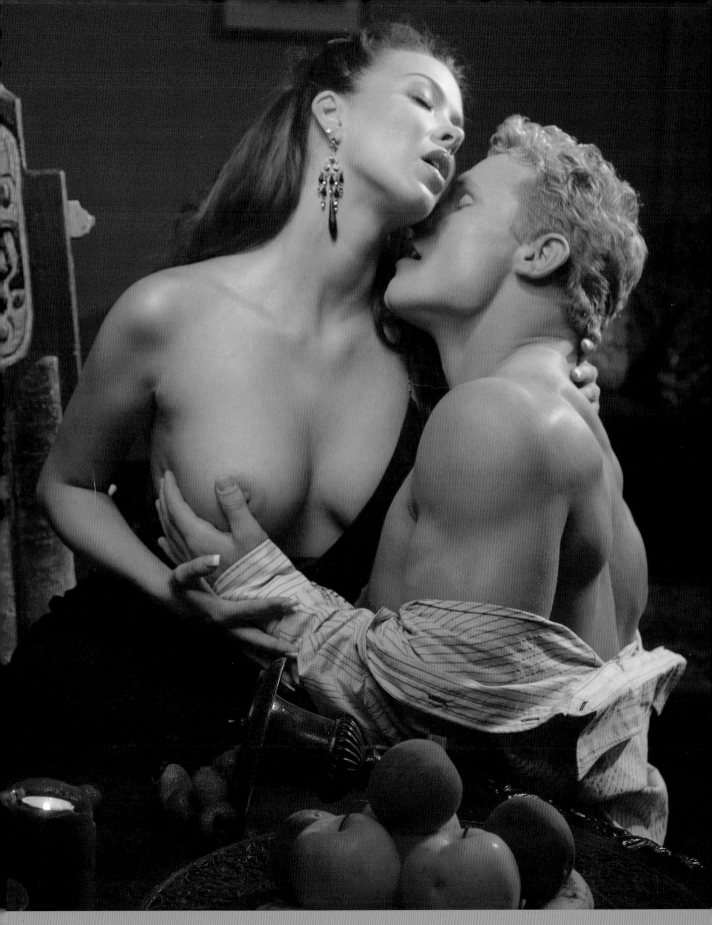

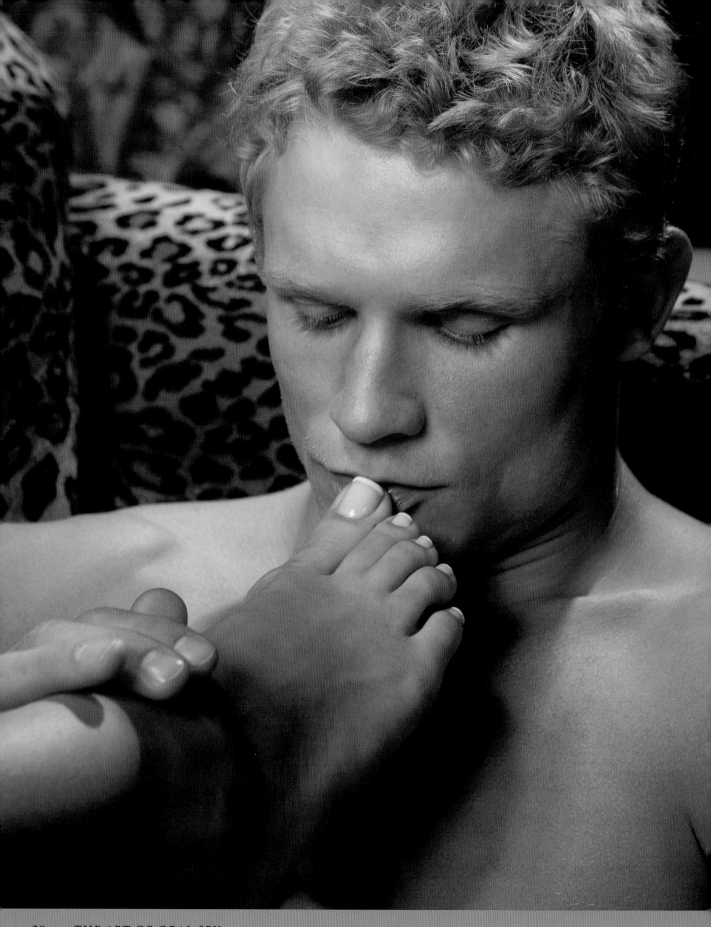

THE SHOULDERS, CHEST, ARMS, AND BELLY

Between 220 and 190 BC, a Rhodian sculptor created the *Nike (Victory) of Samothrace*. One of the most famous Hellenistic statues ever discovered, the sculpture shows the goddess of victory alighting on a ship's prow, her wings spread and her clinging garments rippling in the wind. And though the head is missing, one cannot help but be dumbstruck with the pure physical beauty of this incredible tribute. Indeed, one of the truest testaments to Greek art is the propensity of marble masterpieces displayed throughout the world, specifically the torsos to which they devoted so much detail. The human torso is certainly far more than breasts and nipples and one should give proper attention to the various sensitive areas in this region. The shoulders, armpits, back (especially the lower region), belly, arms, and hands can be every bit as interesting and inspiring as the chest. As with the head and neck, use your hands, mouth, and body to enjoy every inch.

THE HIPS, THIGHS, AND BUTTOCKS

In photography, the best shot is not always the obvious. In an Ansel Adams' photograph entitled *The Tetons—Snake River*, Wyoming's majestic Grand Teton mountain range rises dramatically above the Snake River, as powerful an example of the towering magnificence found in nature as you'll find anywhere. And yet, one might argue that an equally persuasive statement is made in his classic *Close-up of Leaves in Glacier National Park*, where the intricacies and patterns of his subjects are every bit as mysterious, beautiful, and compelling. The same marvelous conundrum holds true with the human body. Whether discovering the peppery variety of colors in an aging scalp or the tingling sensations brought to life with a kiss to the forehead, you should constantly be on the hunt for new areas to explore in, around, and on your lover. So before diving onto your husband's cock or into your wife's juicy vaginal lips, take a few minutes to fondle her butt cheeks or run your fingers between his thighs away from his throbbing member. The sides of the hips, the valley just above the anus, and the soft area just below the genitals can drive your lover into ecstasy before one lick is laid.

THE LEGS AND FEET

Entire books have been written regarding the feet, from fetish obsession (feet being required to reach sexual climax), to mild podophilia (pronounced sexual interest in feet), to sexual foot reflexology, and everything in-between. Rather than continue that tradition, we'll instead simply mention than in your study of your partner's sexual hot buttons, no area should remain untouched. The legs, including the area behind the knee, are not only visually stimulating but loaded with opportunities for arousal.

TANTALIZING TIP

According to the study of sexual reflexology, massage of the inside of the heel directly correlates to the genital area, as does mildly pinching the front and back of the ankles. The two areas are thought to connect to the energy centers in both the vagina and penile area and by massaging certain areas of the feet these areas can be heightened, sexually.

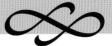

The hamstring area, for example, is highly sensitive and long sweeping strokes from the buttocks to the back of the knee and down to the ankles is not only a huge turn-on, but helps keep the blood circulating for heightened orgasmic potential.

HIS GENITALS

The male sexual organ is as complex as it is misunderstood. No two are alike and they come in different colors, shapes, and sizes. Unfortunately, most modern cultures don't consider the penis a thing of beauty. Add to that the extra burden of media-fueled myths regarding size, homosexuality, staying power, and stamina and it's a wonder men can perform sexually at all these days! Luckily, unadulterated facts (such as the one below), are the most powerful ally in defining a man's sexual potential and enjoyment, as well as the best argument for his partner to embrace his beautiful manhood. After all, in this genre of art, performance is certainly the best indicator of greatness.

THE PENIS

The penis is comprised of two distinct parts. The first is the shaft, which contains the tube (urethra) though which urine flows and drains the bladder. The second part is the glans, which contains the largest number

---

SKIN IS IN!

In *Sex as Nature Intended It*, Kristen O'Hara hypothesizes that penile foreskin is a natural gliding stimulator of the vaginal walls during intercourse, leading to increased clitoral stimulation for more orgasms and in shorter time periods. Heidi Fleiss's father, who is a sexual researcher, believes that male foreskin is akin to a ribbed condom. If either point is true, removal of the foreskin during circumcision might make it more difficult for a woman to achieve orgasm during intercourse.

---

of nerve endings, and is therefore the most sensitive area. Both ejaculate and urine come from the glans. The glans is exposed when the penis becomes erect and is typically where most pleasure, either through oral stimulation or during intercourse, is derived.

THE URETHRA

The urethra is the tube extending from the bladder to the penile opening and is where semen and urine exit the body. These bodily fluids cannot, however, be simultaneously ejected.

THE FORESKIN AND FRENULUM

In the United States, the vast majority of males are circumcised, though attitudes are slowly changing and fewer families are opting for the procedure. In Europe and in other parts of the world, the removal of the foreskin is not as widespread. Circumcision simply means that the foreskin is cut and pulled back

---

DID YOU KNOW?

Don't buy into the bigger-is-better myths. The length of most erect penises is five to five-and-a-half inches (12–14 cm).

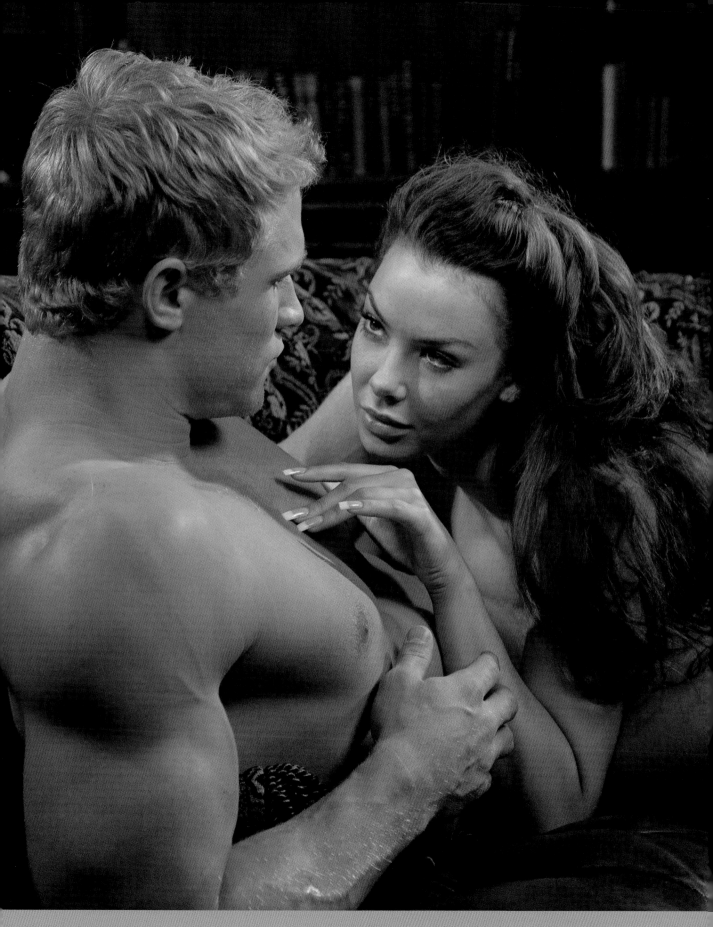

over the glans and frenulum, the tissue responsible for pulling the foreskin back during erection. If you were to base your assumptions on porn films and nude photography, it would be easy to believe males are born this way, but it is not the case. Circumcision dates back to recorded human history, with reasons for the procedure ranging from sacrificial to religious (Islam, Judaism, certain Orthodox Christians) to sanitation (the uncircumcised penis must be kept very clean to avoid infection). The most important factor for you to remember, appearance aside, is that there's very little difference in the sexual performance between the two.

THE BALLS

Underneath the penis lays the scrotum, which is the wrinkly sack containing the testes. Here's where sperm is created and delivered to the urethra, where it will later seek to impregnate its intended target, or wind up gobbled down hungrily by the reader of this book. The all-important cells responsible for the production of testosterone are also located amidst the tangle of tubes. The testicles are an interesting area in that they regulate temperature very efficiently, rising toward the body when seeking warmth and lowering when staying cool. This region is particularly sensitive and many males like to have their testicles stroked, pulled, and even whacked lightly.

THE PERINEUM, ANUS, AND PROSTATE

Behind the testicles, a stretch of skin leads up to the anal opening. This is the perineum, underneath which is the bulb of the penis. Touching this expanse can be quite pleasurable; it becomes hardened along with the male's erection. The anus is rich with nerve endings and can add an enormous amount of pleasure to both oral and sexual intercourse. Once the stigma of touching the area is overcome, a light finger or tongue flicking around the rim or penetrating into the rectum can intensify orgasms in both male and female alike. Further up is the prostate, sometimes referred to as "the male G-spot" for its purported ability to send men into stratospheric heights of ecstasy when it is properly caressed.

TANTALIZING TIPS

- Use fellatio for a healthy heart. In sexual reflexology, it is believed that each area of the genitals corresponds to an organ in the body. Hence, the head of the penis, for example, affects the lung and heart. The clitoris is believed to connect to the kidneys, so on your next trip down, you may in fact be contributing to your partner's overall good health!

- The perineum, the firm area located between the testicles and anus, can be gently pressed during fellatio to help delay ejaculation.

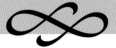

HER GENITALS

The female genital area is divinely matched to its male counterpart, thus enticing the potential sexual partner to join in the creation of life. In addition, the female's anatomy features the *only* body part on either gender whose function is exclusively for pleasure: the clitoris. When studying your subject for creating a masterpiece, never hurry; savor the beauty and wonder before you, perhaps even worship at this temple from which all of us once emerged. Your adoration for her sacred feminine will be rewarded with warmth and shivers.

THE VULVA

The vulva refers to the visible part of the female genitals, which is to say the entire region outside the vagina, including the pubic hair. Pay particularly close attention to the area just between her thighs—blowing, kissing, and touching gently to prepare for further exploration.

THE INNER AND OUTER LIPS

Different on every woman, with varying size, color, and texture, the outer vaginal lips are lined with fat cells, aimed at protecting the vaginal opening and inner areas of the genitals. The inner lips are just slightly below, running the full length of the vaginal opening and covering the clitoris. (They are sometimes aptly referred to as the "hood.") The inner lips end at the perineum, much in the same way the scrotum does on the male. Both sets of lips are highly sensitive, and light blowing to create a chill can be highly arousing. As the inner lips are directly connected to the clitoris, licking them can create high states of arousal and even orgasm.

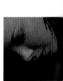

DID YOU KNOW?

- Intercourse isn't the primary way to achieve orgasm for most women; only about thirty percent can climax this way. Most need additional, usually clitoral, stimulation in order to orgasm.

- You should *never* blow into the vagina. Although rare, doing so can result in death by embolism, that is, air being forced into the bloodstream, possibly causing cardiac arrest.

THE URETHRA AND VAGINAL OPENING

The urethra is located between the clitoris and the vaginal opening and functions similarly to the male urethra in that it delivers urine from the bladder out of the body. The vaginal opening is the long tube leading to the cervix, where semen is ushered forward and into the reproductive area for mating with the woman's egg. The vaginal opening can expand to many times its original size to enable a baby to pass through and into the world.

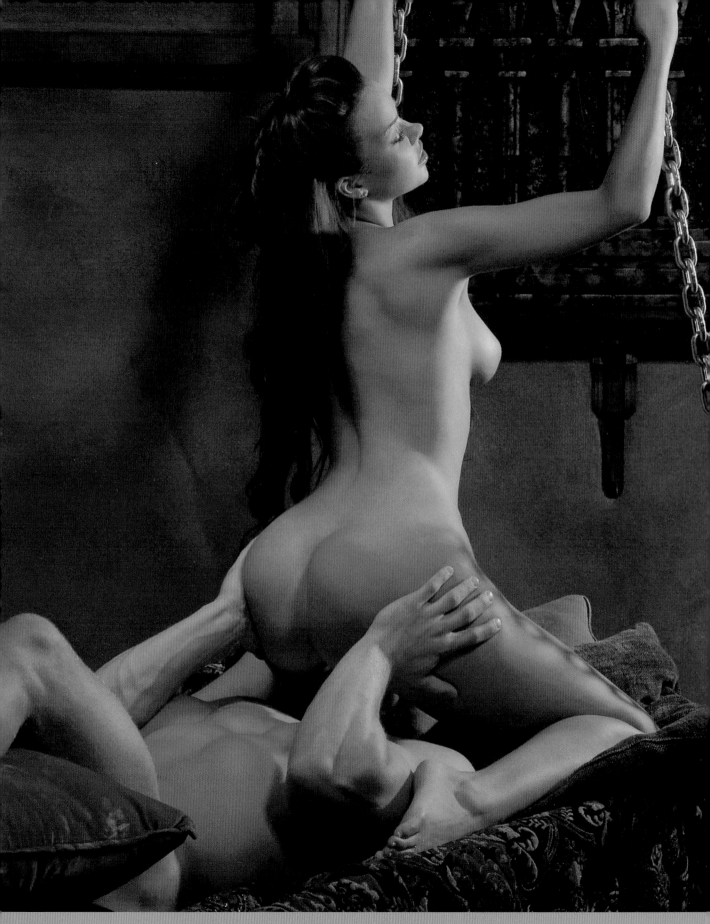

YOUR TONGUE AND THE G-SPOT

Oral sex is the best method to give your female partner a G-spot orgasm! While stimulating her clitoris with your tongue, insert one or two fingers into her vagina, fingers upturned in a hook shape. You only need to insert about half of your finger's length. Feel for a spongy area on the inside wall and press firmly, and then make a "come hither" motion to rub the area. Quicken the pace as her orgasm builds. You will feel the entire inside of her vagina swell around your fingers, meaning her climax is close at hand and she will probably feel the urge to urinate. (It's a good idea to have her use the restroom beforehand.) Make sure you've placed towels down to assure her no mess will be made, and urge her to simply submit to the new sensations. Chances are she'll ejaculate a milky opaque substance that is definitely not urine . . . and your sex lives will never be the same!

THE CLITORIS

The only part of the human anatomy whose soul function is to provide pleasure, the clitoris is the main provider of female orgasms the world over. Covered by the tissues of the prepuce and resting at the crest of the inner vaginal lips, the clitoris remains covered and small until coaxed into action. Once properly stimulated, the clitoris is similar to a male erection, growing up to three times its normal size and engorging with blood to increase its capacity to receive stimulus. In fact, the density of nerve endings in a female clitoris is greater than in any other living creature on earth!

THE G-SPOT

The mythical Grafenberg Spot, or "G-spot," is a controversial subject. It refers to the area just inside the inner wall of the vagina, which is purportedly able to send women into mind-bending orgasms, even resulting in ejaculation, if properly stimulated. There is very little scientific evidence for the existence of the G-spot, although over eighty percent of women believe in its existence, and countless thousands of couples claim to experience G-spot orgasms daily. To reach and stimulate the G-spot, a finger or upturned device is inserted into the vagina and moved in a "come hither" motion. Most women report that this technique, in conjunction with clitoral stimulation, results in higher intensity orgasms.

SEXUAL PLEASURE AND THE HUMAN BODY

Orgasm. Ahhh. That all encompassing goal for sexual initiation, performance, and ultimately, satisfaction. For him, orgasm signifies the passing of his seeds necessary for the creation of life from his body, in essence confirming his entire reason for existing (that is to propagate the human species). For her, orgasm is the single highest physical pleasure for which she's capable—the culmination of several physical and mental processes that result in complete submission to pleasure and ecstasy. When we reach such lofty heights as loving partners, the world seems to melt away around us, wrapping us in the warm glow of love's embrace and filling us with emotions of almost indescribable power.

And yet, what exactly is orgasm? From where does it come? How do we know when we've reached it? And, most importantly, how do we know we've fulfilled our maximum orgasmic potentials?

THE MALE ORGASM

The male orgasm is brought on by rapid, rhythmic contractions of the sphincter, prostate, and muscles of the penis, causing ejaculation; that is, the forced ejection of store semen through the penis's urethral opening, which usually lasts between three and ten seconds.

To achieve orgasm, direct stimulation of the penis and surrounding areas is applied, through intercourse, masturbation, fellatio, or manual device, such as a sleeve. As a man ages, the amount of semen released gradually diminishes, as does the duration of orgasm. However, the pleasure level is usually unaffected. Following ejaculation, it is common for a "refractory period" to occur in which the male cannot achieve another orgasm. This period can vary widely, depending on age, physical health, diet, and other individual factors.

TANTALIZING TIP

Contrary to popular belief, most males can experience multiple orgasms! Through practice and breathing technique, a man can train himself to separate orgasm from ejaculation, which gives him the ability to peak in the same manner as his female counterpart. In their book, *The Multiorgasmic Couple*, Douglas and Rachel Abrams explain step-by-step how men can use Tantric and Taoist principles to go from a one-hit wonder to a platinum performer.

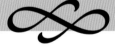

"The tragedy is when you've got sex in the head instead of down where it belongs."

—D.H. LAWRENCE
NOVELIST

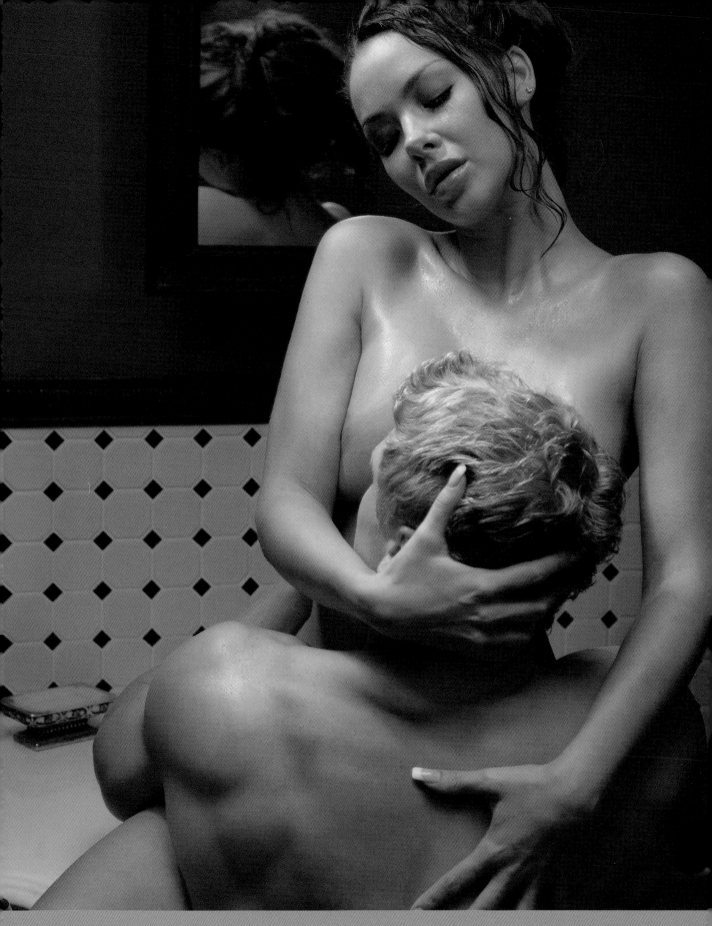

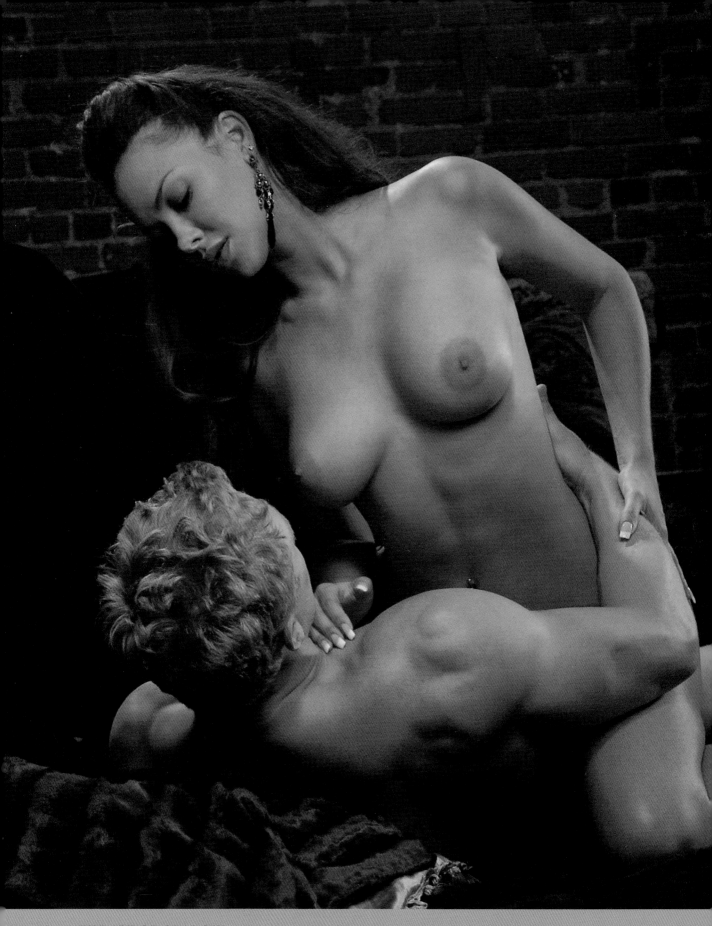

TANTALIZING TIP

The next time you are pleasuring your man with your mouth, keep in mind that, for some men, orgasm continues even after ejaculation. Don't stop just because the ejaculation has stopped. Ejaculation and orgasm are not the same thing and they may not overlap entirely. Ask your partner about his preference.

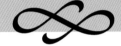

SENSATION

As a man nears orgasm during stimulation of the penis, he feels an intense and highly pleasurable pulsating sensation of neuromuscular euphoria. These pulses begin with a throb of the anal sphincter and travel to the tip of the penis. They eventually increase in speed and intensity as the orgasm approaches, until a final "plateau" of pleasure sustained for several seconds, the orgasm.

During orgasm, semen is ejaculated and may continue to be ejaculated for a few seconds after the euphoric sensation gradually tapers off. It is believed that the exact feeling of "orgasm" varies from one man to another, but most agree that it is a highly pleasurable experience.

PROSTATE ORGASM

Some men are able to achieve orgasm through stimulation of the prostate gland. Men who report the sensation of prostate stimulation often give descriptions similar to women's accounts of G-spot stimulation. Other men report finding anal penetration or stimulation of any kind to be painful, or simply that they derive no pleasure from it. With sufficient stimulation, the prostate can also be "milked." Providing that there is no simultaneous stimulation of the penis, prostate milking can cause ejaculation without orgasm. When combined with penile stimulation, some men report that prostate stimulation increases the volume of their ejaculation. Sperm move at a slow, steady rate from the testes to the prostate where they are ready for orgasm. It is then expelled though the urethra.

DRY ORGASM

A dry orgasm is a male sexual climax that does not result in ejaculation. The term only refers to orgasms experienced by males, as female ejaculation during climax is less common. Prepubescent males are known to have dry orgasms because their bodies are not yet able to produce semen. Males who experience dry orgasms can often produce multiple orgasms, as the need for a rest period, the refractory period, is reduced. Some males are able to masturbate for hours at a time, achieving orgasm many times.

Dry orgasms can be achieved deliberately by putting pressure on the perineum (the beginning of the urethra between the anus and testicles)

DID YOU KNOW?

The average duration of a male orgasm is from three to five seconds; whereas a female orgasm lasts five to eight seconds. Guys on average experience four to six orgasmic contractions at a time; women have anywhere from six to ten.

immediately after orgasm. This causes the urethra to close during ejaculation and thus no semen will leave the penis. This may cause some pain in the testicles and around the anus, and may damage ejaculation-related parts of body including the ejaculatory ducts and vas deferens. Another way to achieve dry orgasm is to, directly after orgasm, contract the muscles used to forcefully stop urination. This can take practice, but men who master it report longer, more intense orgasms, or even the ability to have multiple orgasms.

Dry orgasms may also occur in men who ejaculate multiple times in a short period such as an hour, after the first few ejaculations have used up the available stored seminal fluid. This condition is self-limiting, as after a few hours the supplies of seminal fluid will be replenished by the prostate gland and seminal vesicles.

Men who have had prostate or bladder surgery, for whatever reason, may also experience dry orgasms because of retrograde ejaculation. Retrograde ejaculation is a condition where semen flows into the urinary bladder, rather than through the urethra to the outside.

MULTIPLE ORGASMS

It is possible to have an orgasm without ejaculation (the dry orgasm discussed above) or to ejaculate without reaching orgasm. Some men have reported having multiple consecutive orgasms, particularly without ejaculation. In recent years, a number of books have described various techniques to achieve multiple orgasms. (See page 158 for some recommendations.) Most multiorgasmic men (and their partners) report that refraining from ejaculation results in a far more energetic postorgasm state. Additionally, some men have also reported that this

DID YOU KNOW?

The term "dry orgasm" is also used for a form of mind-body orgasm where the mind experiences orgasm without attempted ejaculation. This type of dry orgasm is one of the goals of Tantric sex.

can produce more powerful ejaculatory orgasms when they choose to have them.

One technique is to put pressure on the perineum, about halfway between the scrotum and the anus, just before ejaculating to prevent ejaculation. This can, however, lead to retrograde ejaculation, that is, redirecting semen into the bladder. It may also cause long-term damage due to the pressure put on the nerves and blood vessels in the perineum.

Other techniques are analogous to reports by multiorgasmic women indicating that they must relax and "let go" to experience multiple orgasms. These techniques involve mental and physical controls over pre-ejaculatory vasocongestion and emissions, rather than ejaculatory contractions or forced retention as above. Sexual energy, though focused in the groin, can be channeled throughout the body. Anecdotally, successful implementation of these techniques can result in continuous or multiple "full-body" orgasms. Gentle digital stimulation of the prostate, seminal vesicles, and vas deferens provides erogenous pleasure that sustains intense emissions

PHARMACEUTICALS, HORMONES, AND THE MALE ORGASM

Internet rumors and a few scientific studies have pointed to the hormone prolactin as the likely cause of the male refractory period, which can contribute to multiple orgasms in men. Because of this, there is currently an experimental interest in drugs that inhibit prolactin, such as Dostinex (also known as Cabeser, or Cabergoline). Anecdotal reports on Dostinex suggest it may be able to eliminate the refractory period altogether, allowing men to experience multiple ejaculatory orgasms in rapid succession. At least one scientific study supports these claims. Dostinex is a hormone-altering drug and has many potential side effects. It has not been approved for treating sexual dysfunction.

Another possible cause of the refractory period may be an increased infusion of the hormone oxytocin. It is widely believed that the amount by which oxytocin is increased may affect the length of each refractory period.

A scientific study to successfully document natural, fully ejaculatory, multiple orgasms in an adult man was conducted at Rutgers University in 1995. During the study, six fully ejaculatory orgasms were experienced in thirty-six minutes, with no apparent refractory period. Later, other scientists observed a single male individual producing multiple orgasms without elevated prolactin response.

Many men who began masturbation or other sexual activity prior to puberty report having been able to achieve multiple nonejaculatory orgasms. This capacity generally disappears with the subject's first ejaculation. Some evidence indicates that orgasms of men before puberty are qualitatively similar to the "normal" female experience of orgasm, suggesting that hormonal changes during puberty have a strong influence on the character of male orgasm.

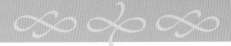

orgasms for some men. A dildo device (the Aneros) claims to stimulate the prostate and help men reach these kinds of orgasms.

Some young men have enough stamina, and may experience sufficient stimulation, that the penis never goes flaccid during the refractory period. Very soon after one orgasm, they may be erect and able to experience another orgasm. Young male children are capable of having multiple orgasms due to the lack of refractory period until they reach their first ejaculation. In female children it is always possible, even after the onset of puberty.

THE FEMALE ORGASM

A human female orgasm is preceded by erection of the clitoris and moistening of the vaginal opening. Some women exhibit a sex flush, a reddening of the skin over much of the body due to increased blood flow to the skin. As a woman nears orgasm, the clitoris moves inward under the clitoral hood, and the labia minora (inner lips) become darker. As orgasm becomes imminent, the outer third of the vagina tightens and narrows, while overall the vagina lengthens and dilates and also becomes congested from engorged soft tissue. The uterus then experiences muscular contractions. After orgasm, the clitoris reemerges from under the clitoral hood, and returns to its normal size in less than ten minutes.

A woman experiences full orgasm when her uterus, vagina, anus, and pelvic muscles undergo a series of rhythmic contractions. Most women find these contractions very pleasurable, but some sexually active women do not.

MULTIPLE ORGASMS

Unlike men, women either do not have a refractory period or have a very short one, and thus can experience a second orgasm soon after the first. Some women can even follow this with additional consecutive orgasms. This is known as having multiple orgasms. After the initial orgasm, subsequent climaxes may be stronger or more pleasurable as the stimulation accumulates. Research shows that about thirteen percent of women experience multiple orgasms. A larger number of women may be able to experience this phenomenon with the proper stimulation (such as a vibrator) and the right frame of mind.

Some women, however, report that their clitoris and nipples are very sensitive after climax,

DID YOU KNOW?

Experts estimate that about forty-three percent of American women are either nonorgasmic or will be nonorgasmic for some significant period in their lives; however, all of these women are capable of reaching orgasm.

and additional stimulation can be initially painful. Taking deep, rapid breaths while continuing stimulation can assist in releasing this tension.

VAGINAL VERSUS CLITORAL ORGASMS

A distinction is sometimes made between clitoral and vaginal orgasms in women. An orgasm that results from combined clitoral and vaginal stimulation is called a blended orgasm. Many doctors have claimed that vaginal orgasms do not exist and that female orgasms are obtained only from clitoral arousal. Recent discoveries about the size of the clitoris (it extends inside the body, around the vagina) complicate or may invalidate attempts to distinguish clitoral versus vaginal orgasms.

The concept of the purely vaginal orgasm was first postulated by Sigmund Freud. In 1905, Freud argued that clitoral orgasm was an adolescent phenomenon, and upon reaching puberty the proper response of mature women changes to vaginal orgasms. While Freud provided no evidence for this basic assumption, the consequences of the theory were greatly elaborated, partly because many women felt inadequate when they could not achieve orgasm

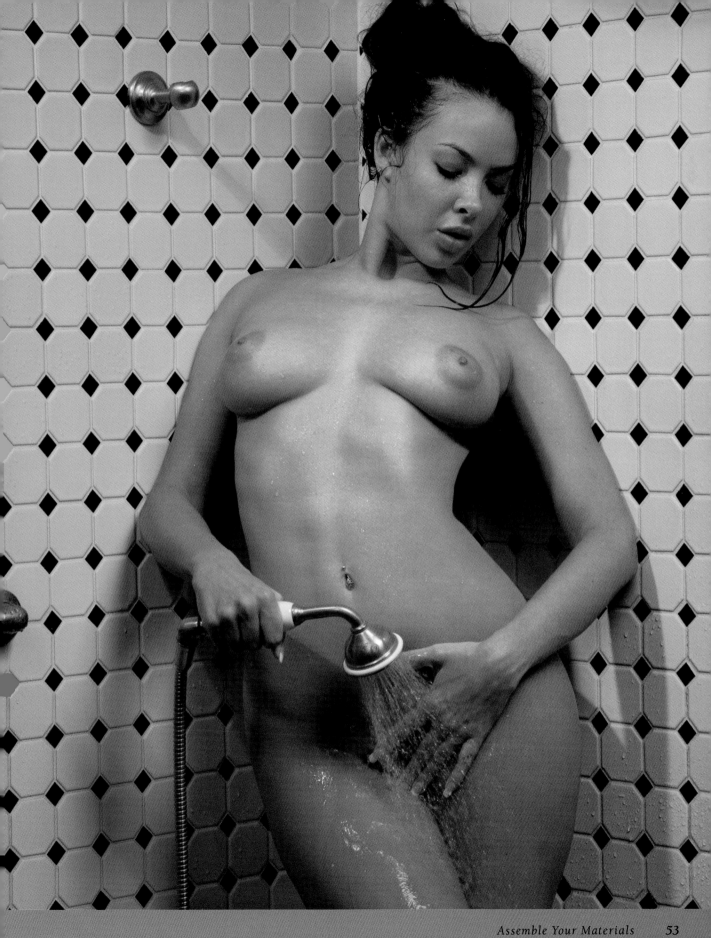

DID YOU KNOW?

A 2005 twin study in Britain found that one in three women reported never or seldom achieving orgasm during intercourse, and only one in ten always orgasmed. This variation in ability to orgasm, generally thought to be psychosocial, was found to be thirty-four to forty-five percent genetic.

via vaginal intercourse that involved little or no clitoral stimulation. Freud's claims about this and many other biological subjects were later largely proven false or based on supposition.

In 1966, Masters and Johnson published pivotal research about the phases of sexual stimulation. Their work included women and men, and unlike Alfred Kinsey earlier, they tried to determine the physiological stages before and after orgasm. One of the results was the promotion of the idea that vaginal and clitoral orgasms follow the same stages of physical response. Masters and Johnson also argued that clitoral stimulation is the primary source of orgasms.

A new understanding of the "vaginal orgasm" has emerged since the 1980s. Many women report that some form of vaginal stimulation in concert with clitoral stimulation is essential to experiencing a fully satisfactory orgasm. Recent anatomical research shows that there are nerves connecting intravaginal tissues and the clitoris. This, with the anatomical evidence that the internal part

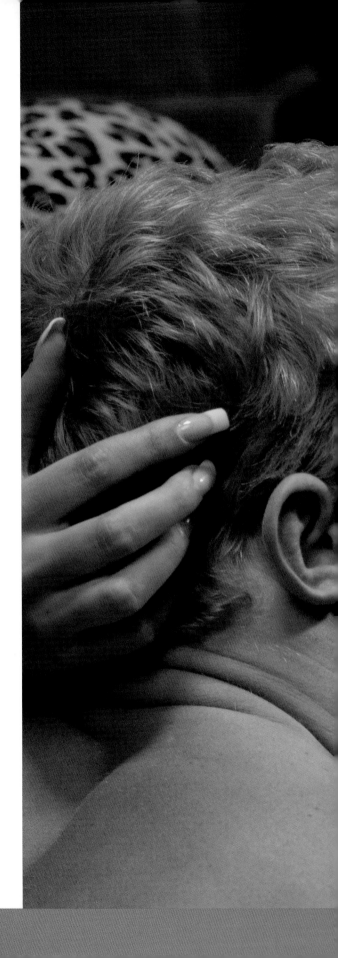

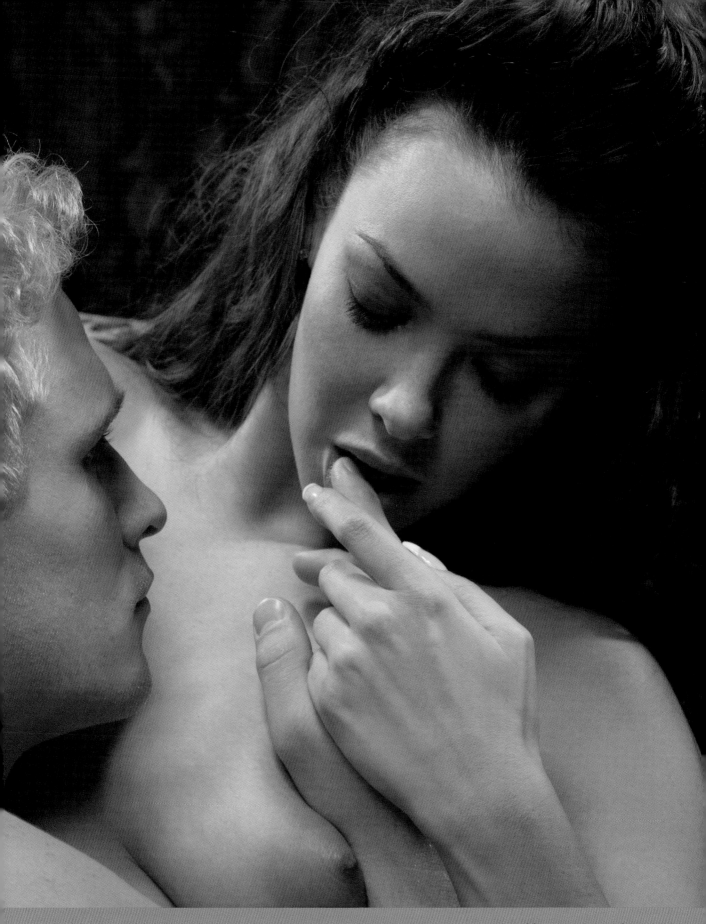

of the clitoris is a much larger organ than previously thought, could explain credible reports of orgasms in women who have undergone clitorectomy as part of so-called "female circumcision" (also called "female genital mutilation"). The link between the clitoris and the vagina is evidence that the clitoris is the "seat" of the female orgasm and is far wider-spread than the visible part most people associate with it. But it is possible that some women have more extensive clitoral tissues and nerves than others, and so that some women can achieve orgasm only by direct stimulation of the external part of the clitoris.

SPONTANEOUS ORGASMS

Orgasm can be spontaneous, seeming to occur with no direct stimulation. Many people find this to be quite embarrassing but enjoyable. Occasionally, orgasm can occur during sexual dreams. The first orgasm of this type was reported among people who had spinal cord injury (SCI). Although SCI very often leads to loss of certain sensations and altered self-perception, a person with this disturbance is not deprived of feelings such as sexual arousal and erotic desires. Thus, some individuals are able to initiate orgasm by mere mental stimulation.

Some nonsexual activity may result in a spontaneous orgasm. The best example of such activity is a release of tension that unintentionally involves slight genital stimulation, like the rubbing of the seat of the bicycle against genitals during riding, exercising, when pelvic muscles are tightened, or when yawning.

It was also discovered that some anti-depressant drugs may provoke spontaneous climax as a side effect. There is no accurate data for how many patients who were on treatment with antidepressant drugs experienced spontaneous orgasm, as most were unwilling to accept the fact.

ORGASM AS VESTIGIAL

The clitoris is homologous to the head of the penis; that is, the head of the penis and clitoris develop from the same embryonic structure. Stephen Jay Gould and other researchers have claimed that the clitoris is vestigial in females, and that female orgasm serves no particular evolutionary function. Proponents of this hypothesis, such as Dr. Elisabeth Lloyd, point to the relative difficulty of achieving female orgasm through vaginal sex, and limited evidence for increased fertility after orgasm.

Feminists such as Natalie Angier criticized that this hypothesis understates the psychosocial value of female orgasm. Catherine Blackledge, in *The Story of V,* criticized the hypothesis from a more scientific standpoint, citing studies that indicate a possible connection between orgasm and conception.

Some nonsexual activity may result in a spontaneous orgasm. The best example of such activity is a release of tension that unintentionally involves slight genital stimulation, like the rubbing of the seat of the bicycle against genitals during riding.

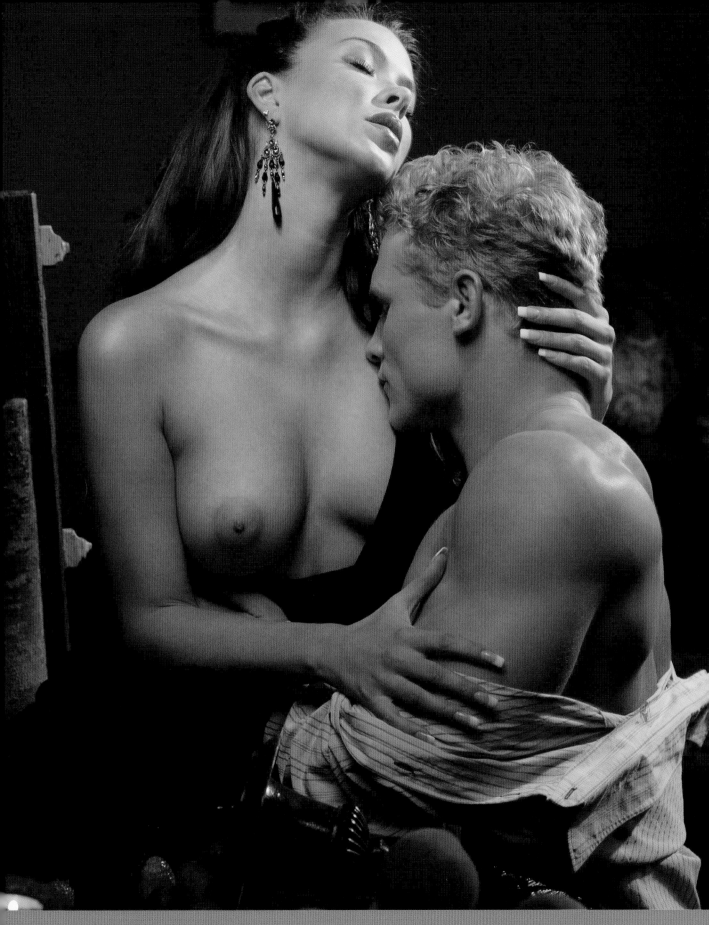

ANAL ORGASM

Anal orgasm is an orgasm brought on by anal stimulation, such as from an inserted finger, penis, or sex toy. Some men and some women are able to achieve an anal orgasm, resulting in a complete or incomplete sexual climax.

A woman may come to orgasm without stimulating the anus, but by stimulation of the buttocks and anal cleft with the tongue. Typically, anal orgasm is brought on by stimulation of the G-spot, through the wall shared between the vagina and the rectum, from a sex toy, finger, or a penis.

WHY DO FEMALES ORGASM?

Evolutionary biologists have several hypotheses about the role of the female orgasm in terms of the reproductive process. In 1967, Desmond Morris first suggested in his pop-science book, *The Naked Ape*, that female orgasm evolved to encourage physical intimacy with a male partner and help reinforce the pair bond. Morris suggested that the relative difficulty in achieving female orgasm, in comparison to the male's, might be favorable in terms of Darwinian evolution by leading the female to select mates who bore qualities like patience, care, imagination, and intelligence, as opposed to qualities like size and aggression that pertain to mate selection in other primates.

Morris also proposed that orgasm might facilitate conception by exhausting the female and keeping her horizontal, thus preventing the sperm from leaking out. This possibility, sometimes called the "poleax or knockout hypothesis," is now considered highly doubtful.

Other theories are based on the idea that the female orgasm might increase fertility. For example, the thirty percent reduction in size of the vagina could help clench onto the penis, which would make it more stimulating for the male, thus ensuring faster or more voluminous ejaculation. British biologists Baker and Bellis have suggested that the female orgasm may have an "upsuck" action (similar to the esophagus' ability to swallow) resulting in the retaining of favorable sperm and making conception more likely.

A 1997 Learning Channel documentary on sex had fiber optic cameras placed inside the vagina of a woman while she had sexual intercourse. During her orgasm, her pelvic muscles contracted and her cervix dipped into a pool of semen in the vagina, thereby making conception more likely. The fact that women tend to climax more easily when they are ovulating also suggests that orgasms are tied to fertility.

Other biologists surmise that the orgasm simply serves to motivate sex, thus increasing the rate of reproduction and helping ensure the species' survival. Since males typically reach orgasms faster than females, it potentially encourages a female's desire to engage in intercourse more frequently, increasing the likelihood of a successful attempt at conception.

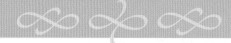

This is often greatly facilitated through additional manual stimulation of the clitoris. Anecdotal evidence suggests that some women experience anal orgasm as qualitatively different from clitoral or vaginal orgasm, though for many others the distinction is less clear.

In both sexes, pleasure can be derived from the nerve endings around the anus and the anus itself. Hence, anal-oral contact can still be pleasurable without stimulation of the clitoris. Anal orgasm has nothing whatsoever to do with the prostate orgasm, although the two are often confused.

SIMULTANEOUS ORGASM

Simultaneous orgasm (also referred to as mutual orgasm) is a sexual climax achieved by partners at the same time during intercourse. It is believed that during simultaneous climax a man and a woman can experience the highest point of sexual satisfaction.

Wilhelm Reich, an Austrian psychoanalyst, suggested in his works that orgasm is more intense if sexual peaks of both partners coincide. This

happens when both partners are able to focus on their sensations as well as emotional closeness with each other. Dr. Alfred Kinsey, a pioneer researcher on human sexuality, emphasized that simultaneous orgasm is the most intense, yet rare, experience a couple can achieve in intimate relationships.

According to the belief that male sexual response is much easier and quicker than the female's, the usual way to reach synchronized orgasm is to delay ejaculation in men and hasten the climax in women. Although many couples desire simultaneous orgasm, it usually results from coincidence and is quite rare. The odds of achieving this lofty goal are, however, greatly increased with proper procedure and timing.

Simultaneous orgasm (also referred to as mutual orgasm) is a sexual climax achieved by partners at the same time during intercourse. It is believed that during simultaneous climax a man and a woman can experience the highest point of sexual satisfaction.

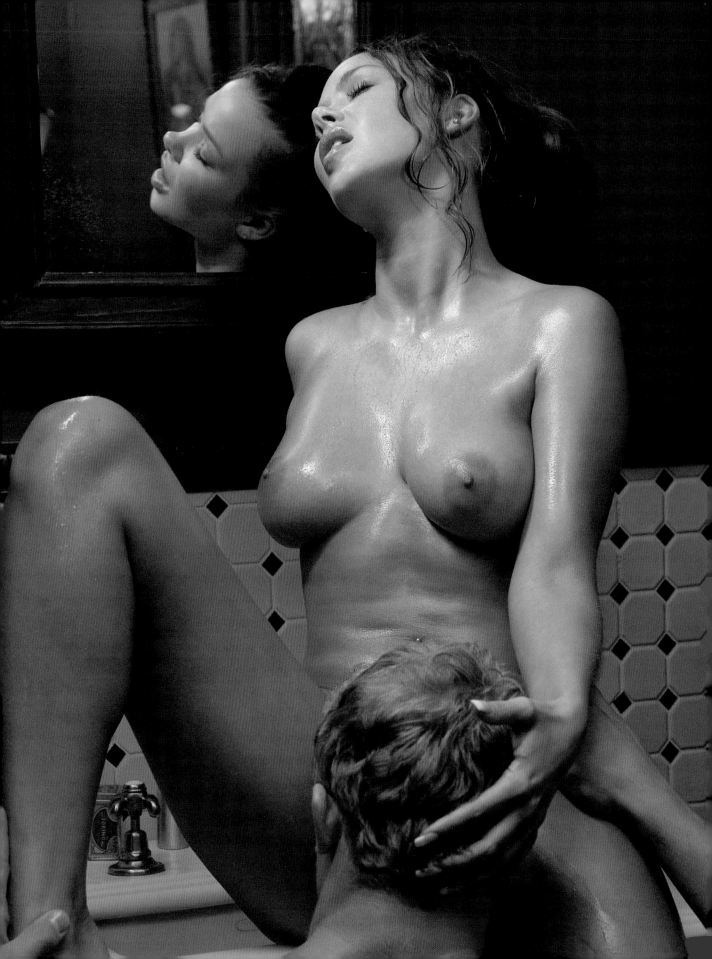

4

THE ART OF PLEASURING HER:
Cunnilingus

"Cunnilingus is next to godliness."

—ANONYMOUS

GREAT LOVERS AREN'T BORN TOGETHER, but they can certainly die together. Becoming a great oral lover takes great practice, patience, trust, and purpose. As Dr. Paul explained in his anecdote (see pages 63–64), it wasn't until he left the lights on and embraced the beauty of his partner's vagina that he could become a true artist in pleasure.

If you view your journeys downward as merely a step closer to plunging your erection into her wet opening, you will never fully realize the amazing satisfaction that comes with giving wholly to your partner's sexual enjoyment. In our own relationship, we view going down as its own separate act, progressing as if nothing else matters. Only by finding your own joy through providing hers will you finally reach the depth of feeling that accompanies basic physical pleasing.

WARMING HER UP

Your first steps should *not* be throwing her legs over your shoulders, sucking her clitoris into your mouth, and attacking it as if you haven't had a bite to eat in months. These types of trysts certainly have their time and place (see Quiver Books' *The Art of the Quickie* for more on this type of thing), but we're talking oral *sex*, not oral velocity. Thus, we recommend you address each section of her body through massage or simple cuddling, avoiding her genital area entirely until she's sufficiently warmed up and ready. (Observing her body language for clues will help let you know when she's good to go.)

Take your time, relax, and let your tongue and fingers slowly glide over her body, teasing and tasting until she quivers and shivers. Too many males try to force their female's orgasm, rather than assist its development and combustion naturally.

TANTALIZING TIPS

There are dozens of effective (and sexy!) positions in which to perform cunnilingus:

- Woman reclining

- Woman on top

- Doggie position

- Sunny side up

- Standing O

See page 95 to learn more about these positions.

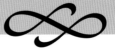

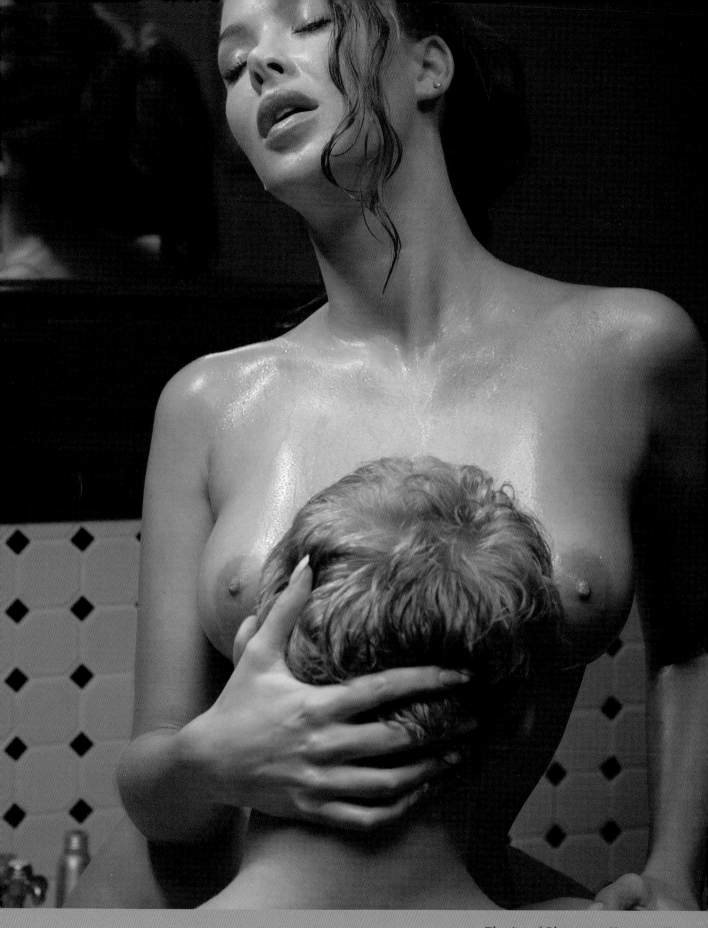

MAKING FRIENDS

Wanting to be a good lover, *I avidly learned from every woman what she wanted and how to please her. I learned how to slowly caress her body, suck tenderly on her breasts and rapidly flick my tongue around her clitoris.*

I even learned to postpone my ejaculation until either she was satisfied or we could attain satisfaction in one gigantic simultaneous explosion. I became a really good technician and very proudly lived up to my reputation with a variety of appreciative females.

Then one time my partner asked me, "How do you like my vagina?"

"It's O.K.," I replied weakly.

"Well, what do you think about when you see my vagina?" she pressed on. "I don't know. I don't think much about it. Since we either make love in the dark or my eyes are closed, I guess I rarely see your vagina."

This line of questioning made me very uncomfortable. Like any good soldier I had always just dutifully kept my nose to the grindstone, so to speak, and patiently waited for that most welcome tap on my head, or other appropriate signal, that told me I could move on to the really good stuff. Even though I was getting pretty uncomfortable, she wasn't done.

"What do you like about giving me head?" she asked.

"That's an easy one," I replied. "I enjoy giving you pleasure."

"I like that too" she purred and, "It would really make me feel good if you really enjoyed it for yourself. Do you think it would increase your pleasure if you saw my vagina as beautiful and as a place that you got great pleasure from for yourself?"

"Sure, but I never thought about it that way."

"Well, next time we make love how about leaving the lights on, keeping your eyes open."

Like any intrepid explorer, as I plunged into the adventure of a whole new experience I started to discover amazing new delights. Really seeing and knowing a woman's vagina became a fascinating journey into the depths of this most enchanting labyrinth of nooks and crannies. With my tongue as well as my fingers, I explored the wonderfully complex contours of her vagina and the

"Well, next time we make love how about leaving the lights on, [and] keeping your eyes open?"

subtle variety of colors that actually changed during
every experience.

Of course, as I became a connoisseur and
loved spending more time with my new "friend,"
the experience opened up new possibilities for my
partner's sexual responsiveness. I had never continued
to suck on a woman's vagina through her orgasm until
I learned to love the vagina. Staying with her through
her orgasm not only allowed the power of her orgasm
to increase, but also provided me with the ride of my
life. Entering her as her orgasm was winding down,
brought new life into her experience and often became
the wonderful way we ended our lovemaking together.
It took me many months before I got up the nerve to
ask my partner the question that pointed us in yet
another illuminating direction, "What do you enjoy
about giving me head?"

Seeing a vagina as a delicate flower also led me
to really appreciate the genius of Georgia O'Keeffe. I
became enthralled with her paintings and one of her
thoughts continues to have a great impact on my life:
"Still—in a way—nobody sees a flower—really—it's
so small—we haven't time—and to see takes time,
like to have a friend takes time."

~ BY JORDAN PAUL, PH.D.

READY FOR ACTION

Once you've adequately lavished attention to her sexy body, your foray into her love nest should be no less caring. In fact, it should be even more so. Once again, slow and steady is the key; before plunging your tongue into her opening, lightly lick the area just inside her thighs. Use your breath to warm and cool each area from top to bottom and then lightly play with her outer lips. The object is to gradually increase her desire, so resist the temptation to head for her clitoris for as long as possible.

After lavishing attention to her outer lips, use your fingers to part them slightly, feeling for her inner lips with your tongue, always slowly and gently. Always be aware that less is more and that the object is to *compel* to her climax, so draw out each step as long as possible: take all night if your tongue and fingers have the stamina!

TANTALIZING TIP

Talk or sing to her vagina. The low hum of your voice will stimulate the entire area and your worship will enliven her senses. (By the way, the same technique works during fellatio—hence, the term "hummer.")

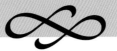

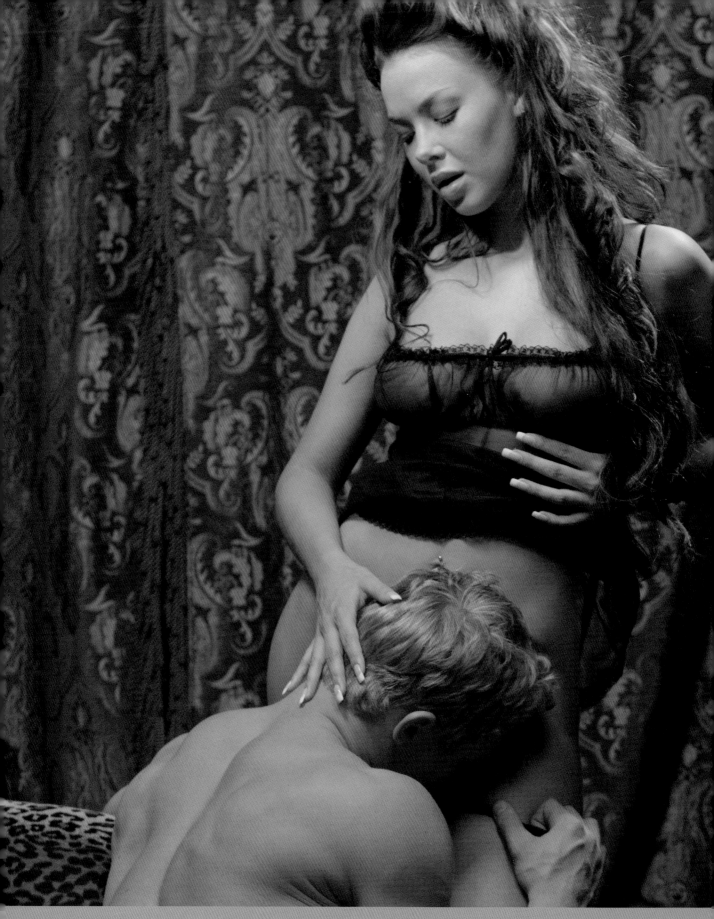

THE EXCITING CLIMAX

By now, her vagina should be soaking wet from the combination of your saliva and her natural juices; this is the time to find your way to her clitoris. Once there, continue to take your time, running your tongue around and over the prepuce (hood), then taking long strokes with the tip of your tongue and lightly grazing the small exposed area of her clit. Use your forefinger to lightly probe the inner lips in a circular motion, inserting only the first digit, while continuing to tease the clitoris from its protective hood. As her clitoris swells, you can use the forefinger and index finger of your opposite hand (in a V shape) to pull back the prepuce, exposing the clitoris fully. Apply light pressure and rhythmic strokes with your tongue, letting her body language guide you toward her climax.

As her orgasm builds, you may wish to begin plunging your fingers into her juicy vagina to emulate penetration or wrap your arms around her thighs to hold her in place as you continue to lick, faster and faster until her eyes roll back and she loses her mind in orgasmic bliss.

Once she's climaxed, bring her down gently with light massage over her lips and vulva, taking time to kiss and revel in the unparalleled beauty of her vaginal area. Feel free to repeat as necessary . . .

"The clit is a tiny cock and the cock is a giant clit, for all intents and purposes. So, to improve cunnilingus in an instant, suck her vulva as you like your not-yet-hard-but-will-be-soon cock sucked. For ladies, I just tell them that if they lovelovelove cocks in general, they'll be able to love this particular one no problem, if they just let themselves sink into the sensual feast that is the man package."*

—NINA HARTLEY
SEX PERFORMER, EDUCATOR, AND AUTHOR

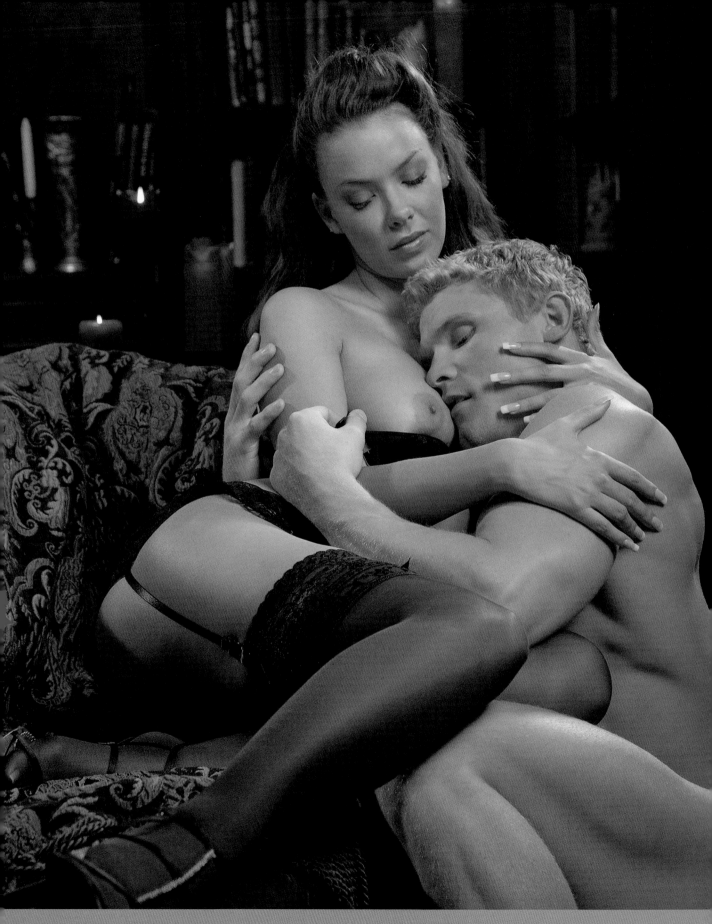

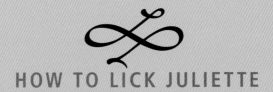

HOW TO LICK JULIETTE

This is a brief lesson in pussy licking that was requested
by a young man lacking in experience who wanted
some "tricks" for the tongue.

The trick is, if there is a trick at all, not just to learn, but
to unlearn every time, with every different person. I don't
know if I buy into the whole thing about having "skills"
and "techniques." My first orgasm was experienced with
a guy who was a virgin. I had been with a few technically
"experienced" guys before him; however, their experience
had merely programmed them with a routine that was not
specific to me: my body, my rhythms, my idiosyncratic little
ass. This guy just went by intuition and paid attention, and
he did a fine job. He figured me out like I was a musical
instrument. There wasn't any pressure, just pleasure. We
simply played around . . . licked, sucked, fucked, groaned,
and giggled until something happened or we fell asleep.

I preface by saying, of course, that I only have
experience with my **own** pussy, so everything I say is my
own opinion. Oh yeah, and all this is off the top of my
head, but here we go . . . Now then, some tips on orally
pleasuring a lady:

Step one: SLOW DOWN!

Everything is all hot and heavy and you get to the
moment and she's gonna let you do it and you drop down
there . . . and then, you STOP . . .

Make her wait a second (just a second), let the body
cool for an instant. You can even gently blow on the pussy.

Spread the lips open. Lick around the lips, nibble on the
inner thighs. Make her want it. Massage the ass. Spread
her open. And then, move in . . .

A strange thing happens when I'm getting licked.
My mind is focused on one thing and one thing only when
it's time to get the pussy licked: the clit. I get absolutely
focused on coming, like that's all there is. Waiting for it,
building up to it, is almost torture. I get greedy and lazy.
I want it and I want it now. Any teasing is a torment. It's
alright, though, because it's all part of the game; and the
better a guy can play me, the better it is. I get taken on
a journey . . . I re-live episodes from my childhood . . .
I go through high-school again. It's a fucking meditative
therapeutic head-trip when it's good. There is nothing in
this world so wonderful at a clitoral orgasm brought forth
by the gentle wet tickle of a soft and talented tongue. It is
fucking amazing. And we love you for it.

If you plummet full-faced into the fray, without
direction, discipline, or attention to detail, the sensation
received is a general, more mental, sensation. The mind
registers something like, "Oh, he's eating my pussy" and
that's about it. When you slow it down, it gets specific.

Continued on p. 70

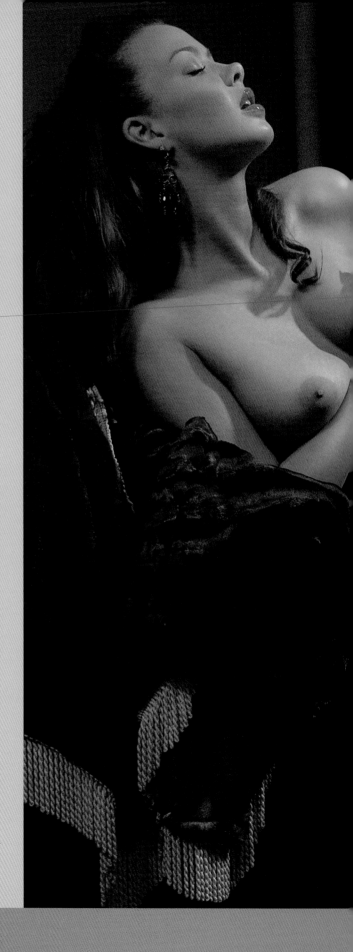

Continued from p. 69

We feel every lick, probe, touch . . . I can feel the air hitting my wet lips when I'm spread open. I'm given the time to shudder and respond to every new sensation. It's not a race, it's an experience. The goal is to learn something new about my body, my self, my capacity to feel.

Now for specific tips! (This is starting to get me all sauced up and crazy.)

When you're fingering . . . full, deep, slow thrusts are often preferable to fast ramming.

G-spot stimulation: find the G-spot! The best way to do this is to move your finger like you're beckoning someone to "come." (Funny coincidence, huh?) The magic spot is toward the front side of the vaginal wall, and when I have a G-spot orgasm while receiving oral sex, I drip like a faucet.

We love it when you eat our asses. We don't judge you for it. You rock if you will shamelessly eat our asses like it's some sort of pie eating contest gone wild. Finger in the ass is good . . . slow and steady, playing my ass like an accordion.

And rhythm . . . slow, steady, building . . . like a good symphony.

Sucking on the clit is sooooo nice; light, light nibbling is nice, and putting a finger in the ass while sucking on the clit (this is the accordion feeling) is mind-blowing.

Let your mind go; let yourself be in the moment. Just flow and go with it. There are times during oral sex that I forget I have a body, and I become a giant, glowing, infinite pussy, pulsing and wet, and the man buried in my juices is like some eight-armed Shiva, doing some mystical dance all over my nervous system. He is a God, and I am nothing but sex.

Oh lord, whatever. Just make me melt and lick up the drippings. I'm gonna go take a shower now.

~BY JULI CROCKETT

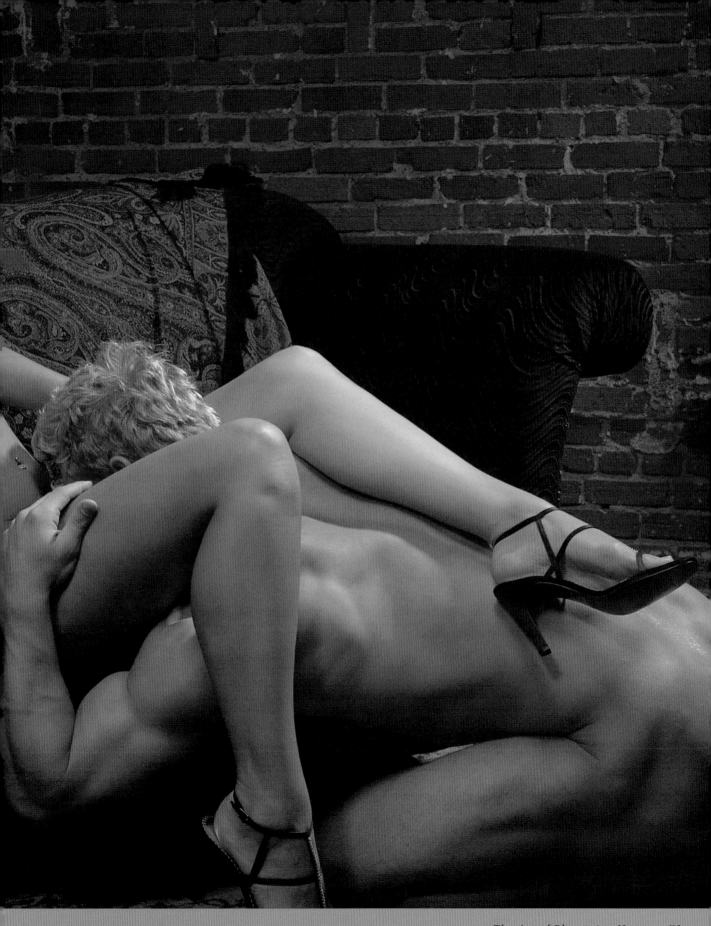

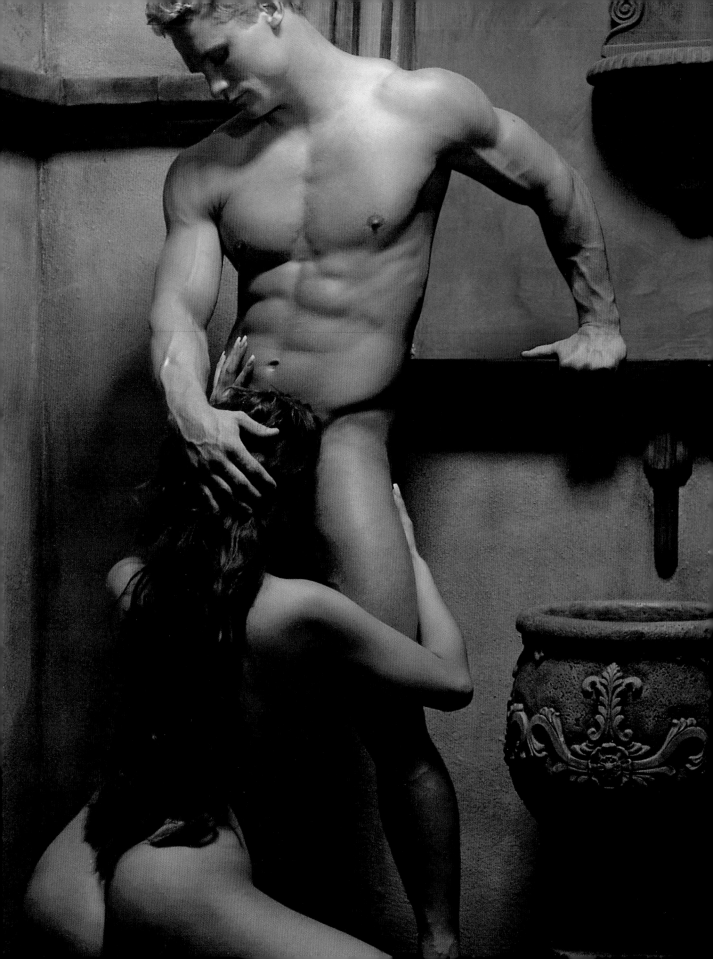

5

THE ART
OF
PLEASURING HIM:
Fellatio

*"Graze on my lips; and if those hills
be dry, stray lower, where the pleasant
fountains lie."*

—WILLIAM SHAKESPEARE

WHY GIVE HEAD?

It may sound naïve, but this is a question we get
asked quite frequently in our day-to-day encounters
with women both single, dating, and in long-term
relationships. Our answers vary. "It's a great way to
substitute for sexual intercourse if you're not ready
to take that step with your partner," is one response.
Other answers are along the lines of "it's just plain
fun," or "because it's a wonderful and giving act."

Whatever the reason, performing fellatio is
an intimate, passionate act that should be approached
with enthusiasm and desire. For the woman, fellatio
puts her in complete control of her man's pleasure,
from beginning to climax. She can challenge her own
oral skills to try to finish him quickly, or draw him
into a long and torturous ordeal, making him beg for
mercy until she grants him his orgasmic wish. For
the male, getting a good hummer is not only pleasing
from a physical standpoint, but gives a sense of
sexual power and dominance that can heighten his
sexual state. As an appetizer to sexual intercourse,
fellatio is a no-brainer and can help him last longer,
akin to the old technique of masturbating before a
hot date to guarantee a longer lasting interlude.

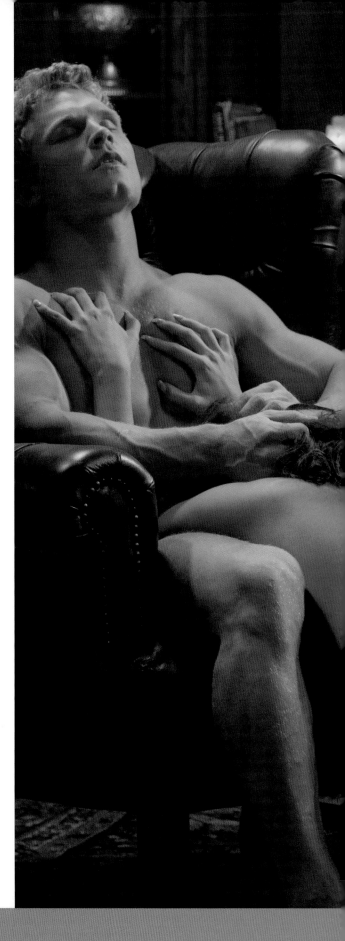

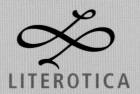

LITEROTICA

"I'm hungry too," *she whispered. Aidan sat up and back until his buttocks rested on the heels of his feet. His dick was pointing straight up.*

"Come on. Get it. Take it, it's yours," he said pointing to his waiting cock. Frieda sat up and slipped the straps of the ruined gown off of her shoulders. She got on her knees and picked up the container of melted chocolate. Aidan grinned knowingly.

"Time for dessert?" he asked.

"Mmmm hmmm," she agreed. She tilted the container and drizzled chocolate over the straight line of his cock, stopping just before it reached the head. She set the container aside and watched while the chocolate ran down the sides of his dick and dripped onto the blanket.

All that chocolate made his dick look like an éclair. Of course one shouldn't have anything so cloyingly sweet for breakfast. But then again, who says? With that thought she preceded to lick the chocolate off of his dick like it was going to be her last meal. Aidan grit his teeth. His wife's tongue could make the CIA give up the government's secrets. Then again, when she finally put it in her mouth, he forgot his own name.

Frieda began to suck him slowly, firmly into her mouth and towards the back of her throat. Each time the head felt like it was going to touch her tonsils, she pulled back, tightening her jaws as she went. She used *her saliva to aid her when she sucked him back in again. She continued that pace until he began to moan and ruin her hairdo with his hands. She then picked up speed and began to massage him with her hand. Aidan was in limbo. Every time she sucked him off, it looked pornographic. He could feel and hear her saliva swishing around his dick like a washer. She looked up into his eyes and moaned to let him know she was enjoying this as much as he was and he almost came in her mouth. Not that she would have minded, but as it was that his legs had started shaking and sweat began to bead on his back, he knew he was close to doing just that. And for once he didn't want to.*

"Baby," he said through clenched teeth. She kept going, sucking harder. He thanked heaven he was on his knees because he might have lost his balance had he been standing.

"Shit . . . baby . . . stop a minute . . . baby . . . damn . . . ssssss . . . hold up," he stammered. She slowed and then pulled him out of her mouth.

"What's wrong?" she asked.

"Nothin' baby," he panted.

~BY SCOTTIE LOWE

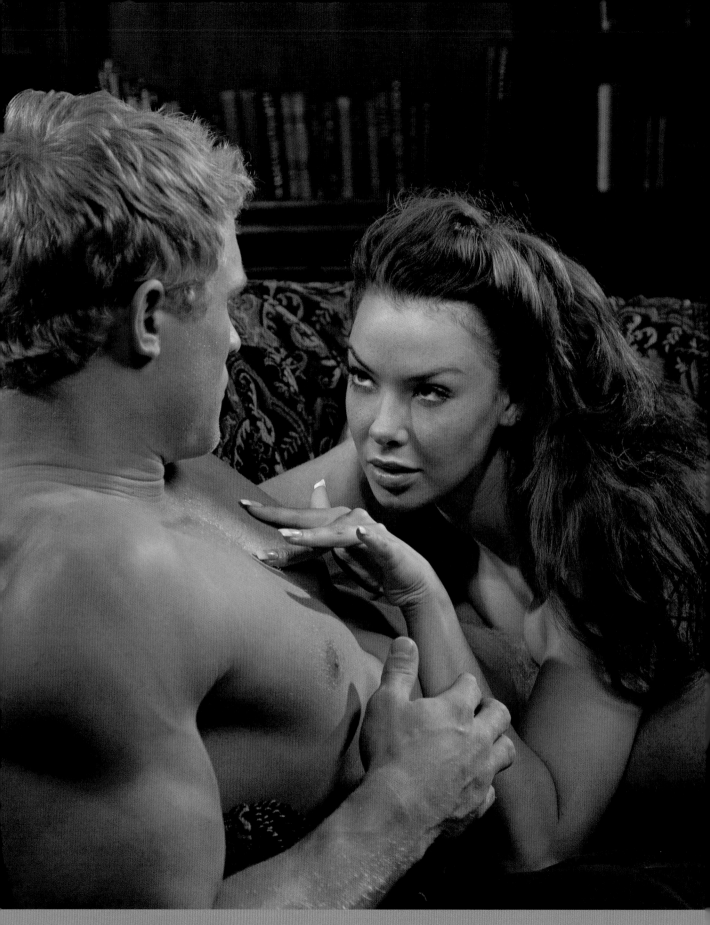

FORGET THE PENIS (FOR NOW)

Too many people concentrate solely on the penis during fellatio. The penis does contain highly sensitive erectile tissue, but there are many other sexually sensitive areas on a man's body. Unknown to many are the pleasures that men receive from having their entire genital area massaged. During oral sex the penis can be stimulated while these other areas are massaged. For example, many men like to have their scrotum and testes fondled or licked during oral sex. Something as simple as placing your hand and cupping the scrotum, or as bold as taking the testes into your mouth, can enhance fellatio to mind-blowing heights.

The most erogenous zones on a man's genitals include the back of the head of the penis (the back being the area leading to his testicles); the line of skin that runs down the center of the testicles, and the underside of the shaft of the penis. Try stimulating these areas with your tongue as well as taking the entire penis into the mouth.

Another form of stimulation that many men like is to have their perineum stroked. The perineum is the area in between the scrotum and the anus. This area is sensitive when the male is aroused. You may like to try rigorously massaging the perineum just prior to orgasm which gives many men a rush of pleasure.

Some men like to have their prostate massaged during oral sex as well. This is accomplished by placing your finger up the man's anus. Make sure that your fingernails have been cut short and place some lubricant on your finger.

Gently run your hand from the perineum to the anus and massage the outside of the anus. Push your finger in the anus with your palm up. Slowly raise your finger until you feel a bump. This bump grows throughout age; it may be the size of a golf ball in young adulthood and the size of a pear in later life. Stimulation of the prostate is an incredible sensation that amazes most men. For maximum effect, apply pressure to his prostate as he's about to ejaculate to intensify his orgasm.

TANTALIZING TIP

As you give your lover head, look up and into his eyes; doing so establishes direct connection and gives the sense you are down there to please. It will drive him wild!

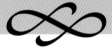

PENIS POINTERS

Now that we've covered the stimulation of the penis' surrounding areas, let's focus on the member itself. Even though the penis is generally sensitive, the majority of its surface area—amazingly—is hardly sensitive to stimulation at all. To give great head, however, the giver must learn about and focus on those targeted areas that *are* the most responsive to sensation.

First on the list is the frenulum, which is the area just under the head and most sensitive to stimulation. The seam, which runs from the base of the scrotum all the way to the head, as well as the base itself, are also quite sensitive to licking and sucking. Focus on each area individually to build anticipation before taking the penis all the way into the mouth.

Once he's putty in your hands and sufficiently begging, you might want to grant his wish and take his member into your mouth. Once you do, however, be careful to keep those teeth in check; contrary to what your impulses may be telling you, teeth and penises do *not* go together. If your lover is abnormally large, try using your lips to cover your teeth (as if you're pretending not to have them at all) and move his penis in and out of your mouth.

During fellatio, lubrication should always be a consideration. Under normal circumstances, saliva will suffice and your mouth will produce more than enough to keep things moving smoothly—especially if your saliva is coupled with his own pre-cum. If you're using a condom during fellatio, purchase UN-lubricated brands and see how things go. If you are unable to produce enough lubrication naturally, look into the various flavored lubricants to help things along (but be sure to ONLY use water-based lubricant products with condoms, as certain substances can break them down).

There are many exciting, sensual, and comfortable positions in which to perform fellatio. See pages 92–93 for some suggestions.

TANTALIZING TIPS

❧ As you go down on him, wrap both hands around his shaft and turn them in different directions. The friction alone will almost certainly finish even the hardiest of lovers.

❧ Size truly doesn't matter. In fact, guys, a smaller penis can actually benefit fellatio by allowing for more of it in her mouth—yummy!

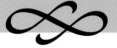

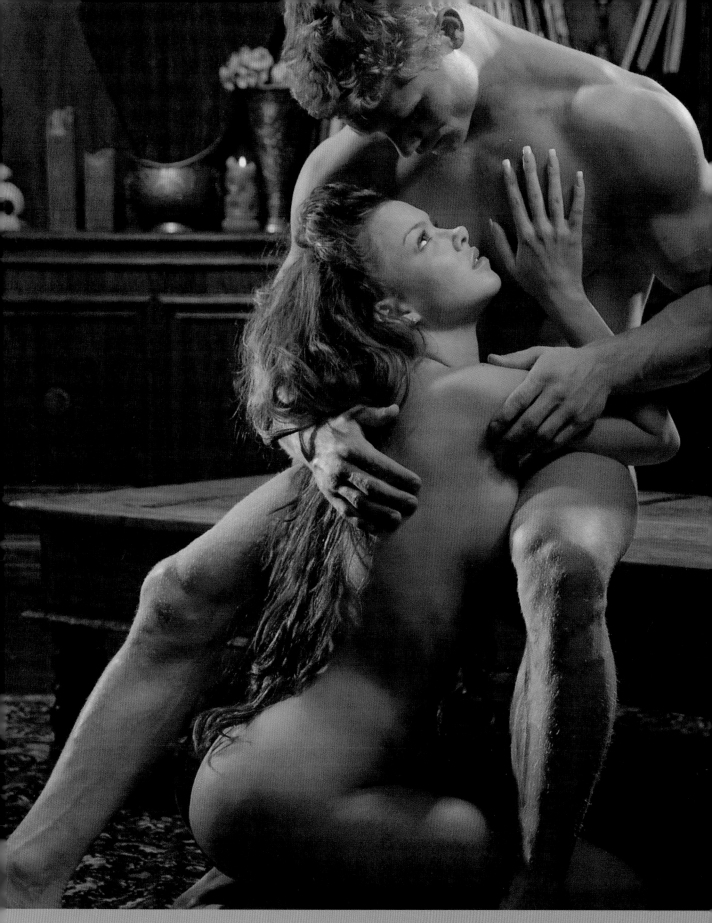

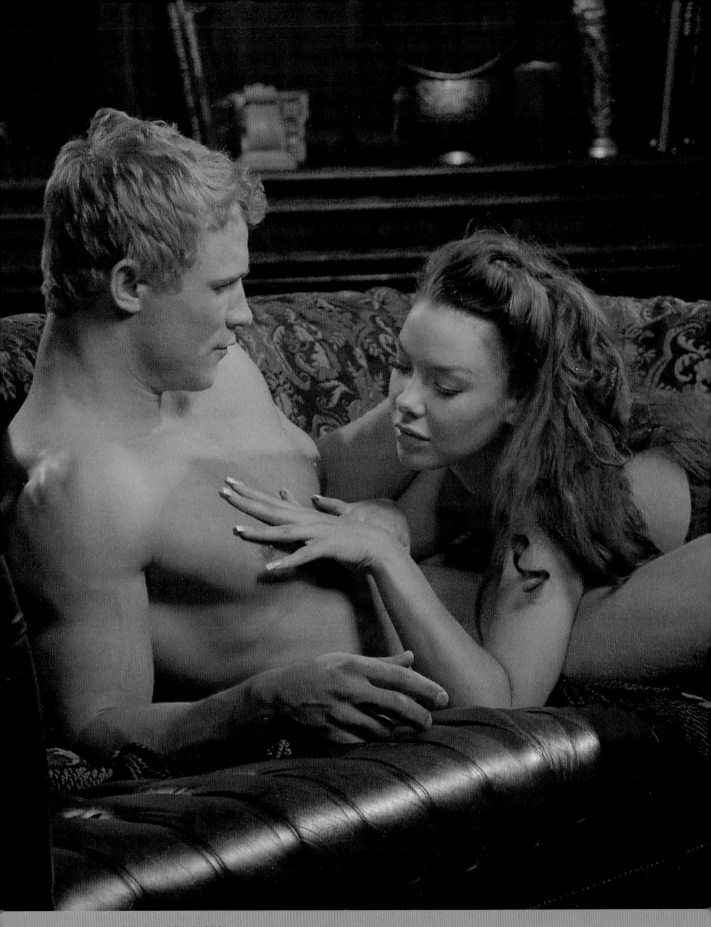

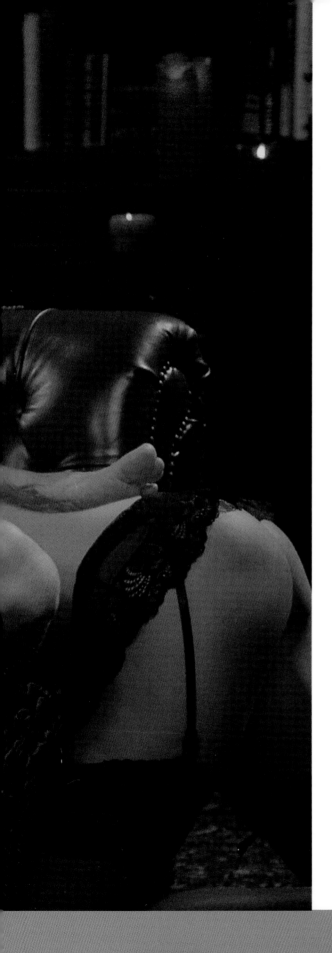

SPIT OR SWALLOW?

So, you've read these tips, and given the blow job of your life. He has ejaculated; what now? Zip up his pants and go shopping? Turn your aroused parts toward his face and receive some reciprocation? There are no hard and fast rules for what to do next, so let your conscience be your guide here. Continuing to lick or suck gently on his flaccid penis is a wonderful way to finish a good blow job. If he's still got some gas in the tank, cuddle up, or mount him and insert his partial erection inside your (probably wet) vagina.

If you've swallowed, it is entirely appropriate to come up from your artistic crouch and issue a long, deep kiss, letting him taste the fruits of your labor. Or simply fondle his package lovingly in your hand until your heart tells you what to do next.

TANTALIZING TIP

Eating a tablespoon of honey or maple syrup (the real stuff) each day can mellow the saltiness of male semen and give a hint of natural flavor.

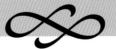

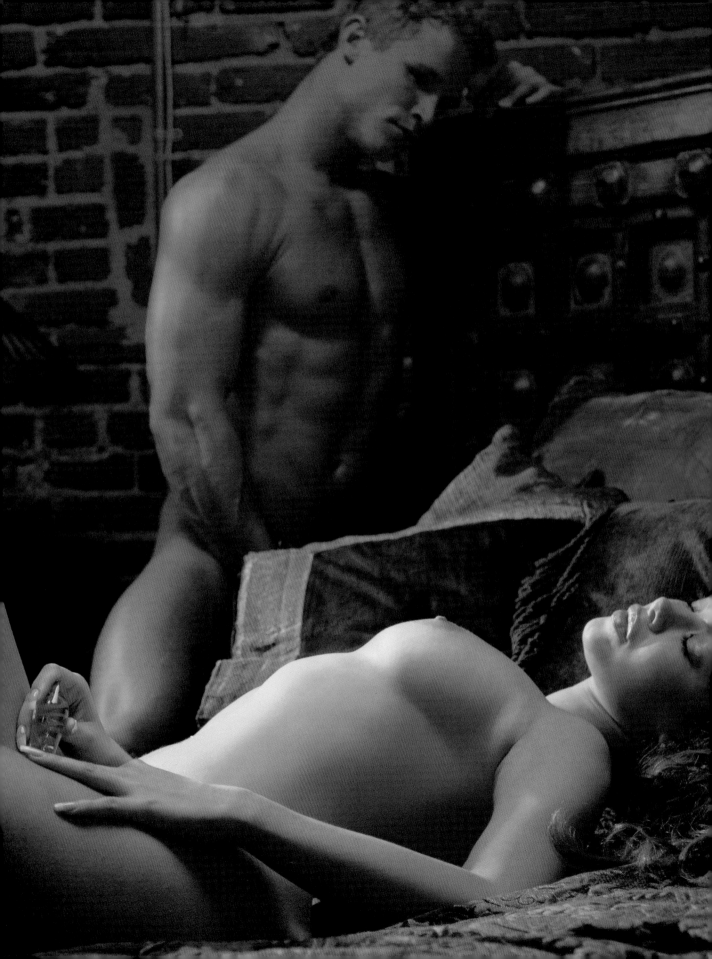

6

THE ARTIST'S TOOLS:

Sex Toys and Aids

"If a man can't handle seeing his lover use a vibrator, my advice to the woman is: keep the vibrator and recycle the man."

—BETTY DODSON, Ph.D.
SEXOLOGIST AND AUTHOR OF *SEX FOR ONE*

NO PHOTOGRAPHER IS CONTENT with one lens, no painter with one brush, nor any sculptor with one chisel. Likewise, no lover should be satisfied with producing sensual art with only his or her immediate tools. Like adding a dash of color to a black-and-white drawing, using a well-placed dildo, vibrator, or masturbation sleeve can greatly increase your orgasmic potential and keep your extremities rested if things progress further. Here are a few tools and tricks no oral artist should ever be without.

VIBRATORS

Adding a vibrator to oral love play is a great way to excite multiple areas simultaneously, as well as provide more intensity to the clitoris than a tongue or finger can. Choose a vibe that is small (or has a small tip), is easy to maneuver, and has multiple intensity settings. The Fun Factory Layaspot, Lelo Lily, and Eroscillator are all fabulous toys to enhance oral play and can be found in most sex shops or online.

DILDOS

Insertable dildos are another fabulous accessory to your artistic palate when savoring your lover's genitals. Available in an almost infinite number of sizes, colors, shapes, and textures, a good quality dildo can come in handy when your fingers begin to tire, or when trying to stimulate that elusive G-spot.

When shopping for a high-quality dildo, pay close attention to the materials; stay away from the cheaper latex and jelly models, as they contain substances that may cause allergic reactions and will begin to deteriorate after only a few months. Medical-grade silicone (found, for example, in products from Tantus) makes sex toys completely inert, meaning they're safe for both vaginal and anal play. They're also nonporous, meaning no bacteria can creep inside.

Glass and metal products are also gaining in popularity for their safety and beauty. The Njoy Pure Wand is a good choice in metal, and glass items from Farenhite Glassworks offer a myriad of oral options.

DID YOU KNOW?

The perineum, the area between the anus and testicles, is highly sensitive and is a terrific place to stimulate during oral play. Apply a small vibrator to the perineum as you perform fellatio to add a little razzamatazz.

TANTALIZING TIP

Don't just run out and buy a dildo on your own; make a date to visit a sex shop and pick one out together. You also might discover new treasures with which to liven up your sexcapades.

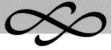

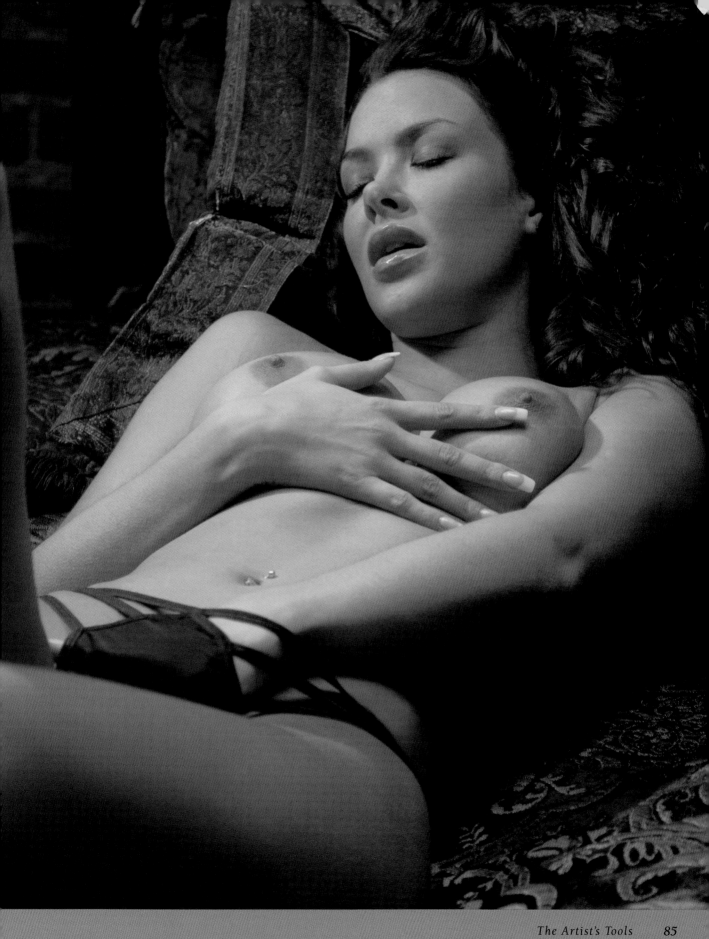

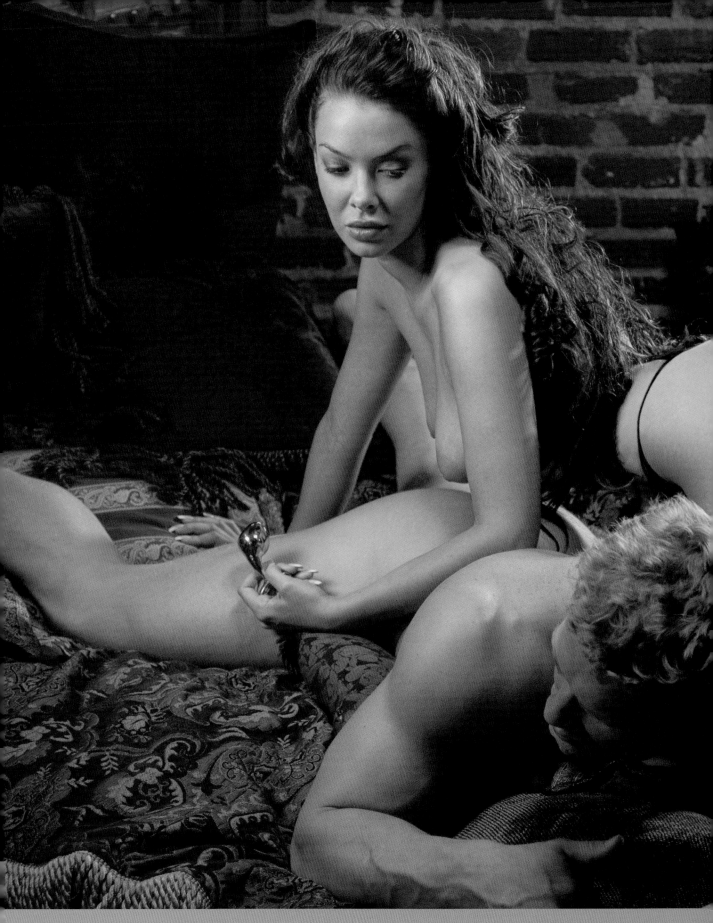

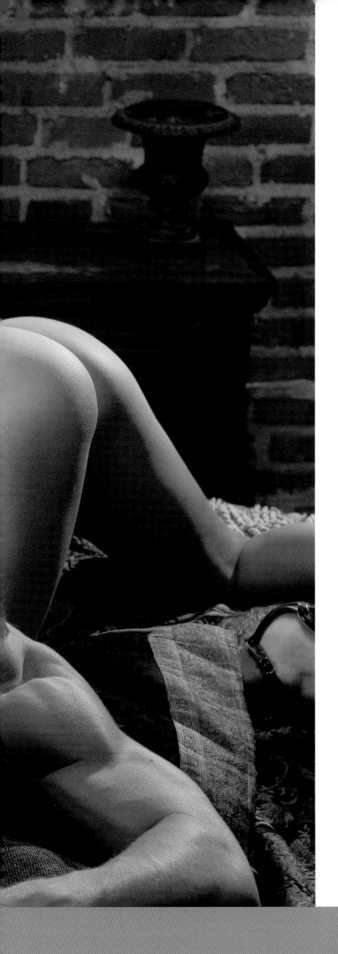

TOYS FOR BOYS

Unfortunately, the traditional adult toy market for males has mostly consisted of the usual XXX-rated videos. Very few items have been offered to specifically enhance *his* sexual escapades; that is, outside of cheaply-made replicas of porn-star mouths and vaginas. Lately, however, male sexual horizons have been expanding, and the adult market is responding with a huge selection of products geared toward improving and/or enhancing his climax.

Cock rings, which trap the blood inside the penis once erect and help to keep an erection longer and harder, are now becoming more elaborate and beautiful. Metal rings from Gear Essentials, for example, are crafted from high-quality stainless steel and can be worn "24/7," ready to fulfill their duties whenever the need arises, so to speak.

Masturbation sleeves, such as the Fleshlight, Vibratex Sidekick, and Hot Rod are made to envelope the penis and mimic the sensations of a real vagina, only tighter. These toys, used in conjunction with a partner's warm, wet lips, will have his orgasms soaring into new dimensions.

HOW TO WEAR A COCK RING

Cock rings come in many different materials and are made to be worn behind the testicles and over the shaft. To use one properly, make sure the area is shaved (you don't want to tug out too many hairs: ouch!) and that your penis is *not* erect. If using a stretchy ring, with two hands pull it as wide as possible and start behind the balls, bringing the ring slowly to rest on top of the shaft. Do not wear stretchy rings for more than twenty to thirty minutes at a time (think of a rubber band around your finger), and make sure to remove the ring if any discoloration or discomfort occurs.

With metal rings, proper sizing is important, so try the following to determine which size is right for you. Wrap a string or thin strip of paper around the entire package (behind the testicles and over the shaft) and divide the total length (in inches) by three and a half to arrive at the proper diameter. To wear, pull one ball through the ring, then the other, and fold the head of the penis down and through the top of the ring. Pull the ring gently back against your abdomen and strut your newly decorated jewels in front of your lover.

ANAL AND PROSTATE STIMULATORS

Whether performing fellatio on him or cunnilingus on her, remember that the anus is packed with nerve endings just waiting to be aroused. And though many of us are squeamish about having our rears stimulated for a variety of reasons (both cultural and sanitation-wise), an incredible opportunity to push our sexual boundaries is being missed by avoiding this fertile area.

If the thought of a finger in your partner's anus doesn't exactly float your boat, there are many

TANTALIZING TIPS

❧ The male prostate, also referred to as "the male G-spot," is sometimes located too far up for fingers to reach. Use one of the many available prostate stimulators to unlock the pleasures in his inner rectum.

❧ Anal stimulation can greatly add to the oral experience. Use your finger to lightly probe the anal opening – use plenty of lube and make sure not to use the same finger in her vagina – and watch her pleasure potential soar to impossible heights.

❧ To expose his anus, have him lay on his back with a pillow or cushion underneath his lower back and buttocks. Push his legs backward, back toward his chest, and apply lube liberally.

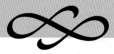

devices designed to stimulate the area that will keep your fingers clean and your mind at ease. Anal plugs, for example, can be purchased in sizes ranging from three-quarters of an inch (2 cm) and up to accommodate just about any comfort level. Prostate stimulators, such as the Aneros, can be used to caress the male prostate and provide consciousness-losing climaxes. As with dildos and vibrators, purchase only products made from nonporous materials, such as silicone, metal, glass, or stone.

ADULT VIDEO

Adult films are not only wonderful mood enhancers, but can also offer plenty of useful techniques and tricks for maximizing your next trip down. In addition to the hot screen sex, most adult movies contain at least three or four scenes of blow jobs and cunnilingus performed by professionals who are paid to make giving head look like an act we'd either like to perform, or have performed. One fun porn game we play now and again is to follow the oral action ourselves exactly as it happens on screen. As the starlet goes down on the male lead, or vice versa, we do the same, precisely emulating the strokes, speed, and method up on the plasma.

ALL ABOUT ALTOIDS

Chewing some mint-flavored candy prior to going down on your partner can add some sizzling sensations to her clitoris. Menthol can provide a new twist on clitoral stimulation, so add a few Tic Tacs or Altoids to your mouth and lightly blow to chill—and then heat—her most sensitive love button. Many topical clitoral creams are also available containing menthol that you can apply for longer lasting effects. (Some guys like it too!)

There are also many educational titles available on DVD that offer explicit instruction in oral pleasure using real-life couples to demonstrate. Those from Alexander Institute and Sinclair are some of our favorites.

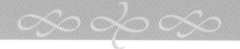

One fun porn game we play now and again is to follow the oral action ourselves exactly as it happens on screen.

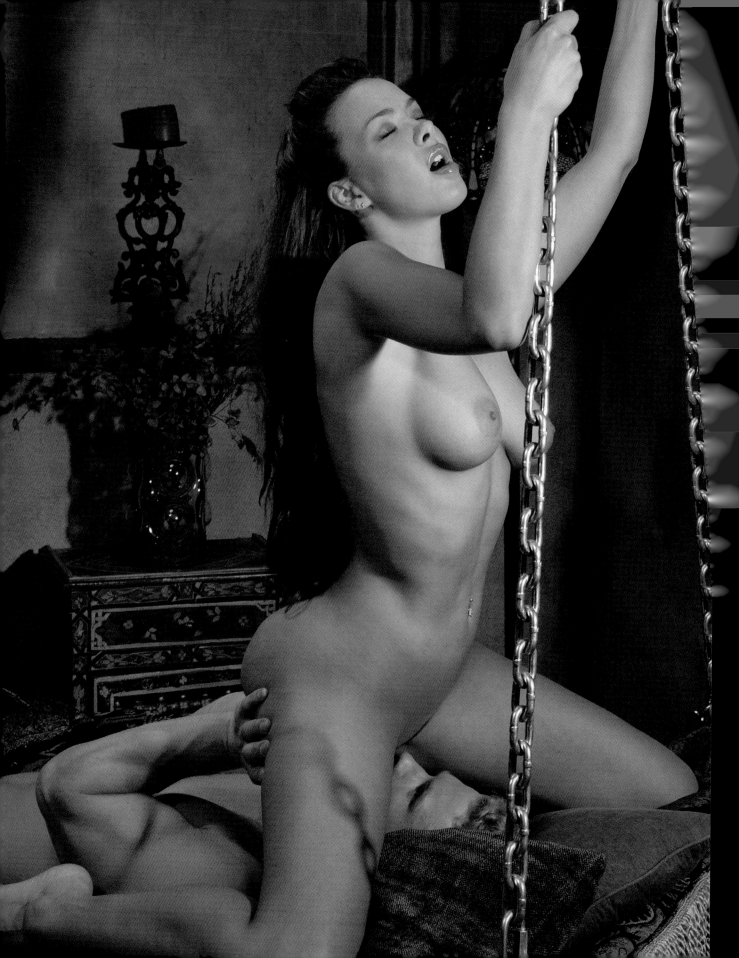

7

ARTISTIC SPACE AND FREEDOM:

Places and Poses for Going Down

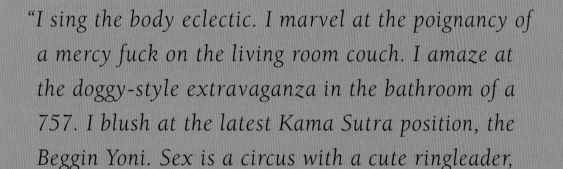

"I sing the body eclectic. I marvel at the poignancy of a mercy fuck on the living room couch. I amaze at the doggy-style extravaganza in the bathroom of a 757. I blush at the latest Kama Sutra position, the Beggin Yoni. Sex is a circus with a cute ringleader, a virtual Chinese restaurant of choices . . . "

—CYNTHIA HEIMEL
AUTHOR OF *SEX TIPS FOR GIRLS*

ALTHOUGH IT'S TEMPTING to assume that the art of going down feels good in any position (okay, that's true enough), there are certainly more optimal positions for keeping heads, necks, and backs out of the chiropractor's office.

The primary focus in oral pleasure should be on comfort for both parties, so if bad knees are an issue, perhaps it's better to find an arrangement that takes the pressure off your tender joints. A bad back? Hunching over her vulva in a subcompact car might not be the best idea. Don't be afraid to change things up either; moving with your mood and flow of sexual progression keeps things exciting and fresh. Most men lie flat on their backs to enjoy fellatio, but there are so many other options to try. Here a just a few.

FELLATIO POSITIONS

STANDING

Incredibly versatile in terms of locations it can be performed, the standing fellatio position is a large part of every man's imagined ideal life. The receiver simply stands or leans against a wall while his partner performs oral sex on him from a kneeling position. Judging from the number of adult films that feature this position, it must be a popular one. The position offers also great access to the receiver's scrotum and anus, if he is okay with some anal play.

Pillows can come in handy with standing positions when the woman is kneeling. Not only do they cushion her knees, but also they can add height, to bring her mouth to the same level as his penis.

SITTING

This position is the most common way to orally pleasure a man and for good reason; it combines two of men's greatest pleasures—sitting and watching. Only, instead of the NBA Finals, he gets a show SO much better! Simply put, the male sits back while the female kneels and "goes down." Nothing fancy, just head-bobbing, mind-blowing action.

Men, use your free hands to either lightly "palm" your lover's head to control her movements on your erect cock, or lightly push her hair out of the way for a clearer view.

THROAT THRUSTING

This can be a very exciting position for many men, and it's especially good for deep throating. The performing partner lies back on a bed tilting her head upwards over the edge while he penetrates her mouth from a kneeling, squatting, or standing position. Make sure you give your lover a break now and again in order to take a breath!

OTHER OPTIONS

There are many other positions that lend themselves to fellatio, such as both partners lying on their sides, using pillows to prop up her head. Also try the male seated in a chair while she crouches down. The main thing to keep in mind is to constantly shift and experiment, finding what's most comfortable, sexy, and fun for both of you.

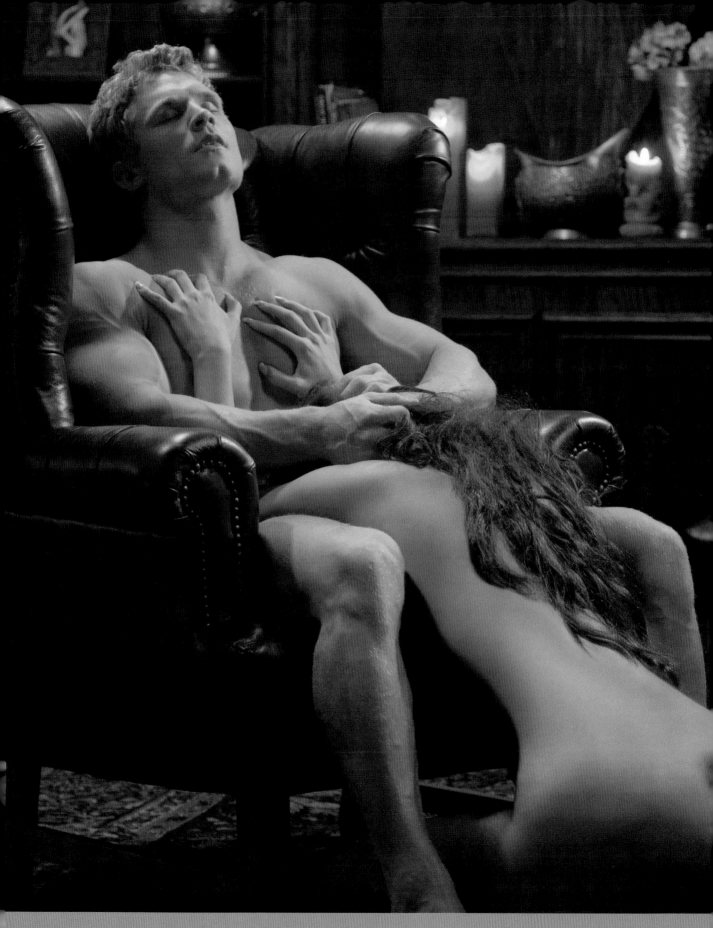

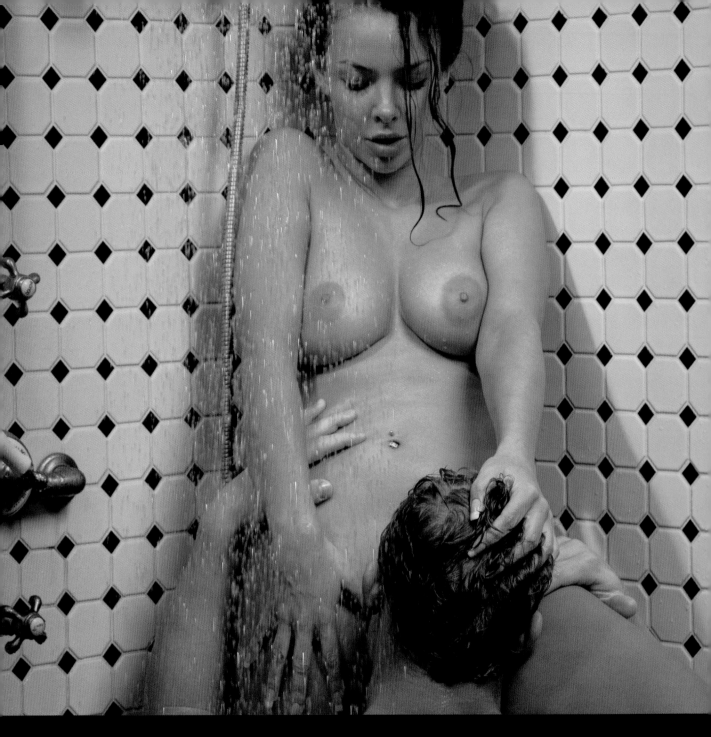

"*The art of life* lies in taking pleasures as they pass, and the keenest pleasures are not intellectual, nor are they always moral."

—ARISTIPPUS
GREEK PHILOSOPHER AND FOUNDER OF THE
CYRENAIC SCHOOL OF HEDONISM

CUNNILINGUS POSITIONS

WOMAN RECLINING

This is the most common position for orally pleasuring a woman. Simply have her lie back and spread her legs. Pleasure her while either kneeling and bending over, or while lying flat on your stomach. Prop her head up with a pillow or two so that she can enjoy watching your oral prowess. Pushing her legs back toward her shoulders exposes more of the erotic areas, including her anus, and is very useful for inserting a toy or two.

WOMAN ON TOP

The man on lies down on his back, and the woman straddles him, her vagina resting over his head and mouth. This position is ideal for her to control her own pleasure, as she is able to move her pelvis to suit her desired angle and speed. For additional comfort, she can lean back, placing her hands on his thighs, which will tilt her pelvis slightly upward, exposing the lower vaginal area and anus. Another variation on this great position is to lean slightly forward and use the headboard for leverage.

DOGGIE POSITION

The doggie position (her on top and standing), whereby she raises her lovely self to receive his oral offerings, gives great access to her anus and is certainly one of the most stunning positions, visually. The female can also "sit on his face," allowing her to control her own pelvic movements (and by extension her own orgasm), much in the same manner as having her on top during intercourse. She can use the headboard for stability as her partner reaches around and upward to stimulate her nipples as she rides his tongue.

SUNNY SIDE UP

With the male laying on his back, the female lays on top of him in the opposite direction, with both partners facing upward. Using a pillow to prop up the male's head, the female slides into position, making for easy access to her anus and vagina. This is a great starting point to eventually assume the 69 position, as the female need only roll over to achieve it.

STANDING O

The male lover lays on his back, head hanging over the edge of the bed (or other surface, such as a table or large couch). The female then straddles over his mouth, moving her hips to the position that feels most pleasurable. This pose is great for females who wish to control the action (and therefore their own orgasms). Be careful not to overdo it, though, as this position can get uncomfortable for the male after too long.

OTHER POSITIONS

Standing is a wonderful way to begin a cunnilingus adventure, as well, and we always enjoy the seated position with the male kneeling down.

TANTALIZING TIP

The next time he is going down on you, use a small vibrator to buzz your clitoris while he fingers you. Guys, use your mouth to keep her lubricated.

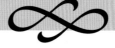

69 POSITIONS

WOMAN ON TOP

In this position, the female is atop the male, facing in the opposite direction. A pillow or cushion propping up the male's head will help prolong cunnilingus by preventing neck strain as he reaches upward to access her vagina.

MAN ON TOP

Similarly to the woman on top position, the male kneels over the woman, his head buried between her thighs and his penis dangling over her mouth.

STANDING 69

Make sure your man has a sturdy back for this one! This advanced position involves lifting the female lover upward, her legs and thighs jutting upward, her mouth in line with his genital area.

SIDE BY SIDE

This variation is probably the most comfortable, due to the reduction of strain on both participants' heads, necks, and shoulders. Lie side-by-side and rest your head on the inner thigh of your partner.

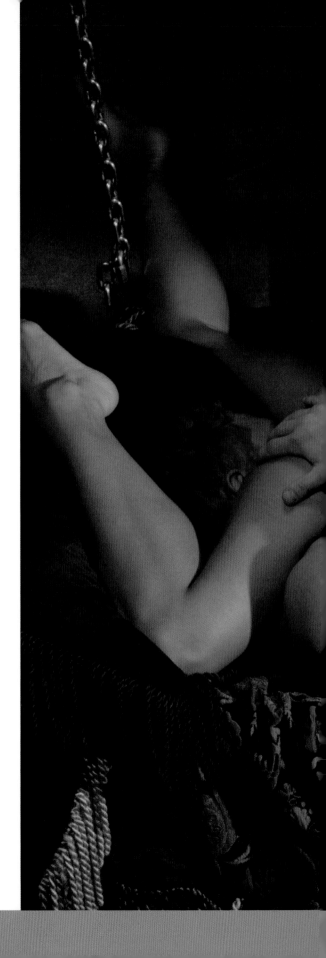

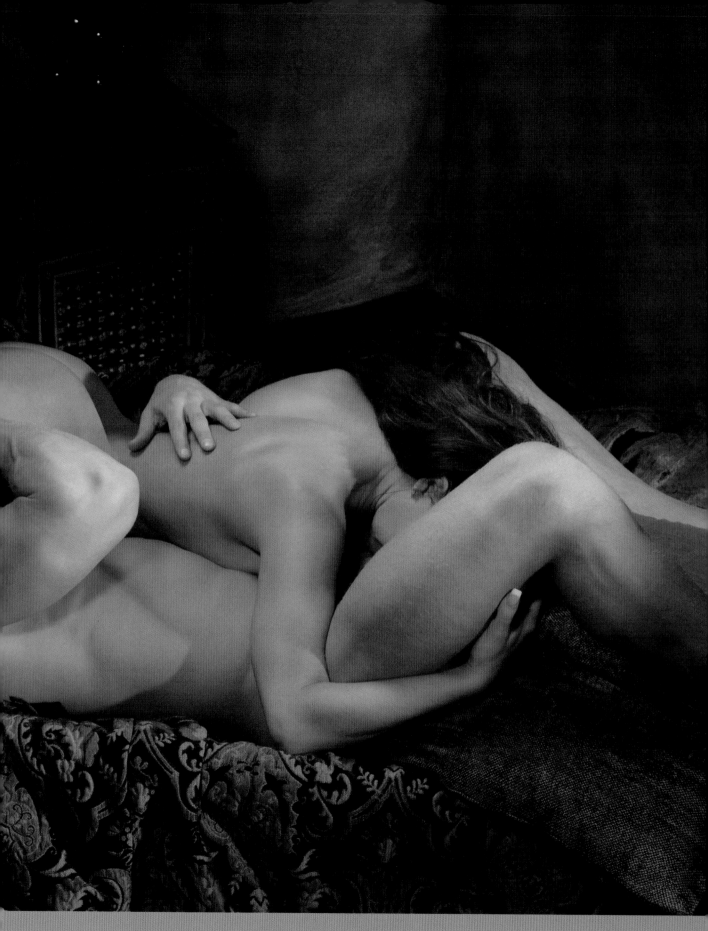

POSITION AIDS

Countless devices are now available to make virtually every facet of love-making more comfortable and easier. Chairs, cushions, suspension apparatuses, and elaborate strap contraptions are designed to put you in positions optimal for oral play, while taking the strain off of your ligaments, joints, and tendons. Sure, pillows are nice, but with a few specialty pieces of sexy equipment, your oral possibilities will be practically unlimited.

LIBERATOR SHAPES

With wedges, ramps, cubes, stages, and their specially-designed Esse chair, the folks at Liberator have come up with a fun and nonthreatening melding of form and function. Made from sturdy foam and covered with velvety smooth fabrics, each shape is crafted to last a lifetime and provide numerous options for sexual positioning.

The simple "Wedge," for example, raises the pelvis approximately six inches (15 cm) to help open the vaginal area by comfortably pushing the legs to

the rear. Exposing her genitals in this manner gives her lover far more access to the area and enables each participant to enjoy cunnilingus for longer periods. If your urge to engage in intercourse interrupts the oral proceedings, simply have her flip from her back to front and enter her easily from behind. The "Ramp" is a superb tool for fellatio, as the male can reside at a relaxed angle to take in all the sights of his partner's oral prowess.

Best of all, the covers of these items are removable and get softer with each wash!

TANTRIC CHAIR

At the higher end of the positioning spectrum is the "Tantra Chair," hand made by ZenByDesign. A long sweeping set of curves with one side higher than the other, this gorgeous item is meant to integrate seamlessly with any living room or bedroom. A multitude of colors and patterns are available to suit most tastes. The chair itself allows for many different oral sex alternatives and is especially effective for deep throating his penis. It is also a nice place in which to engage in sexual meditation together, engaging your sensual minds and bodies into a heightened state of awareness and connection.

SWINGS

The "Love Swing" (and its many imitators) is a suspension device that hangs from the ceiling to provide weightless sexual potential. Made of sturdy nylon straps with padded seat and leg straps, a person inserts his or her legs, sits back, and floats approximately three to four feet (1–1.5 m) off the floor. The adjustable straps enable the swing to be

DID YOU KNOW?

Avoid mixing anal and vaginal fluids! When playing with her anus, either cover your finger with a condom or plan to wash your digit immediately with antibacterial soap before returning to her vagina. Nasty infection can occur when bacteria from the anus enters the vagina, so always play safe.

LOCATION, LOCATION, LOCATION

Don't limit your oral excursions to the bedroom or living room sofa. Your backyard, the side of the road, an empty parking lot, the restroom of a smoky club, just about anyplace is fair game for going down. Use your imagination and don't be afraid to be spontaneous!

Just a few of the places we've given each other oral satisfaction are department store changing rooms, a gas station restroom, an alley behind a former apartment building, every inch of our car (including a convertible with the top down on a busy street), the back of a San Francisco bus, on a Ferris wheel, under a pier in Santa Monica, in a crow's nest at a local park, at a baseball game, in a Maui rain forest, and even on the roof of our house. And although exciting, we don't recommend performing fellatio on the driver of a moving vehicle. (Okay, it's true . . . we tried it ourselves and it was HOT.)

Remember that keeping the sexual sides of ourselves exciting means constantly looking for opportunities to stretch our boundaries. Always be on the lookout for your next unique setting.

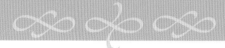

raised or lowered depending on the activity, meaning it's perfect for couples of differing heights.

For oral sex, one simply needs to adjust the height accordingly, depending on the position, and the receiver can relax and enjoy the sensations. For the advanced, the Love Swing can be used to *give* oral pleasure, but we only recommend such extravagances to seasoned lovers.

THE BONK'ER

The Bonk'er is the invention of Jordan Dawes, a Venice Beach, California local artist, who after suffering a broken leg during a soccer match needed a way to elevate his leg during love making. Using his heart as his guide, he shaped two metal lengths into beautiful curves and mounted them on pedestals easily slid between his mattress and box spring. The result is a positioning device with all the

TANTALIZING TIP

Try this. The male is in the standing position, with his partner on her knees. She holds her head still as he thrusts his penis in and out of her mouth slowly, as if engaged in intercourse. This mock-intercourse allows the male to control his movements and bring himself to climax, leaving her hands free to roam his body.

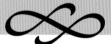

functionality of a sex swing but without the hassle of navigating beams and difficult setup. Indeed, either partner can sit or lie within the Bonk'er and experience weightless (and effortless) oral sex.

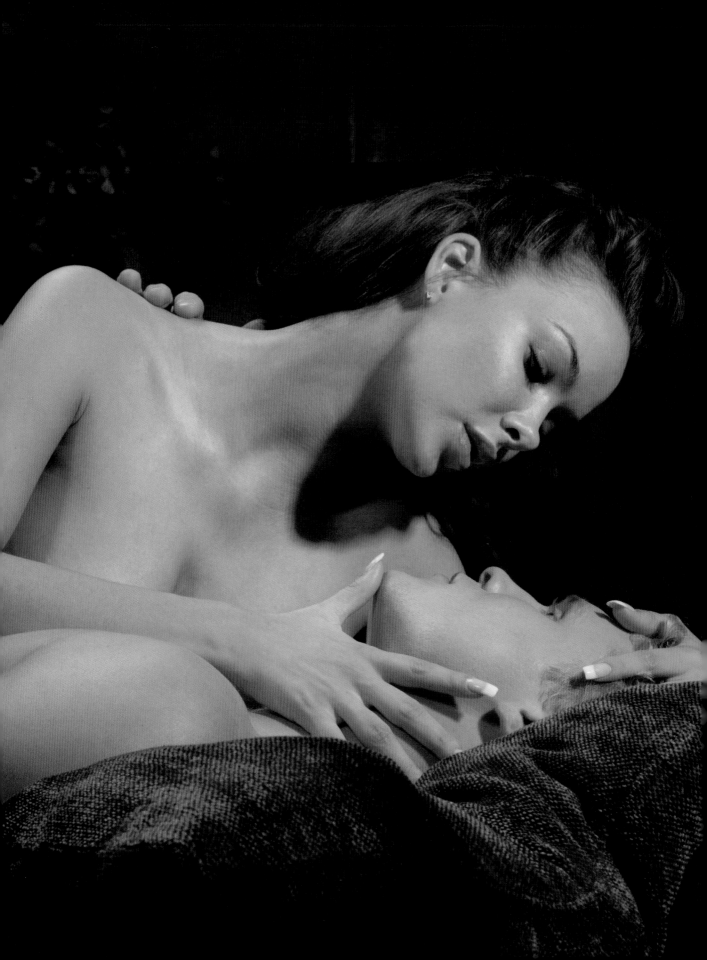

8

ARTISTIC LICENSE:

Protection and Expanding Your Repertoire

"I regret to say that we of the FBI are powerless to act in cases of oral-genital intimacy, unless it has in some way obstructed interstate commerce."

—J. EDGAR HOOVER
FORMER DIRECTOR OF THE
U.S. FEDERAL BUREAU OF INVESTIGATION

PROTECTION

Remember the Clinton defense? That going down can somehow be categorized as something other than "sex?" We instead harbor the belief that any practice involving the exchange of intimate body fluids pretty much qualifies as meeting the adequate definition. Hence, it's important to point out that STDs (sexually transmitted diseases) *can* be passed through oral play. If you at all unsure about the status of your lover's sexual health, have him or her visit a doctor before going anywhere near the genital area. At the very least, use a condom for fellatio or gloves for cunnilingus if you are the least bit hesitant.

When using condoms for the prevention of STDs, avoid latex or animal skin, as they are porous and can assist in transmission of certain diseases.

DID YOU KNOW?

Several diseases (some more serious than others) can be transmitted through oral sexual activity. Among them are gonorrhea, hepatitis A–C, herpes, syphilis, lice, crabs, chlamydia, and HIV.

Better to choose polyurethane and those without spermicidal additives. Many condoms are now available in pleasant flavors to address the taste issue.

SPIT OR SWALLOW?

For the first eight years of our marriage, the thought of her swallowing a load of fresh male cum didn't appeal to either of us. Apparently, we're not alone: countless emails and personal stories shared on our website and in person in our adult store confirm that a large percentage of females recoil in horror at the thought of swallowing a load of salty egg whites.

For some, it's a texture aversion; in others the taste is the issue; and, in rare instances, safety concerns, such as the fear of receiving an STD, are at the root of the problem. From the male perspective, watching her run to the bathroom sink or immediately reach for a towel is not the ideal way

to cap a great blow job. If the thought of swallowing your partner's fluids dampens your enthusiasm, try having him ejaculate further toward your throat, which will avoid having the taste on your tongue. Another way of overcoming the swallowing issue is to keep a soda or glass of juice nearby, washing his love juice down with a quick swig.

Or do what the porn stars do; have him come in your open mouth and let it run back out and down his shaft, using the slickness to stroke his penis for one last moment of bliss. In our case, we took baby steps. She swallowed only small amounts at first, then gradually took more and more until the whole load

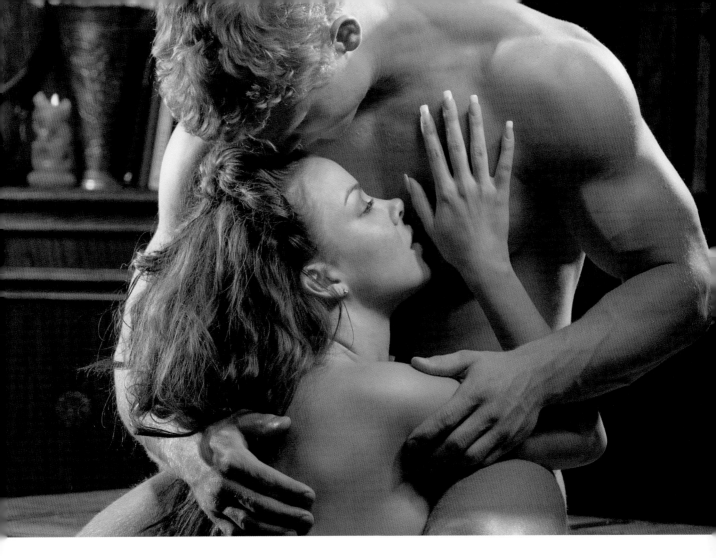

went down without a hiccup. Eventually, we grew to love the act of swallowing so much, that it's not uncommon for us to now pull out during intercourse at the instant of climax and finish off with a healthy gulp.

If, however, nothing works for you, and swallowing just isn't an option, there are alternatives. As mentioned previously, letting your lover ejaculate only partially into your mouth, then letting it run down his shaft is one alternative. Another is to position yourself so that he can release onto your breasts or another sexy part of your body—perhaps using your hands for the final few strokes.

TANTALIZING TIP

Men, when it "comes" to swallowing, what's good for the goose, as they say, is good for the gander. A good method to get her more comfortable with swallowing (or taking your cum in her mouth in general) is to stop her during her licks on your dick to kiss her. (Or kiss her immediately after you've ejaculated in her mouth.) Letting you know your own fluids don't disgust you can go a long way toward gaining acceptance in her mouth on a regular basis.

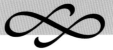

DEEP THROATING

In 1972, the movie "Deep Throat" was released, dramatically changing both the porn industry and the way oral sex would forever be perceived. Starring a young woman named Linda Susan Boreman, who went by the stage name Linda Lovelace, the film was about a young, sexually frustrated woman, whose clitoris is "discovered" to reside in the back of her throat. Only by having a penis reach deeply into her throat could she experience orgasm, sending Lovelace on a "prescription" to perform deep throat on men until finding one suitable to marry. Estimates vary, but there are claims the film has grossed over a billion U.S. dollars since its release, making it not only one of the highest-grossing movies of all time, but a testament to the popularity of the fellatio act itself.

Since an average erect penis is longer than the depth of an average mouth, deep-throating requires suppressing the gag reflex in order to partially swallow the end of the penis. To perform this form of fellatio, the giver controls all the muscles at the back of the throat and flattens the tongue, while gradually inserting the erect penis completely.

In a variation of the technique, the woman lies face up on a bed, with her head hanging over the edge. For some fellators, this ensures that the throat and mouth line up, aiding penetration, and can also give the fellatee additional control over the act, which may be desirable if the couple is experimenting with domination and submission play.

Because mouth and throat structure (as well as penis shape) vary from person to person, different persons will prefer different techniques and positions, and some experimentation may be necessary.

Deep throating may facilitate swallowing of the semen, as the ejaculate often bypasses most of the tongue and taste buds, depending on the depth of penetration at the time of release. If the penis is held completely inside the mouth and throat as the man ejaculates, the semen may be released into the esophagus without the receiver having to swallow.

Additionally, many men enjoy the sensations and psychological effects associated with the act. Similarly, many women and men enjoy incorporating it into their sexual repertoires, particularly as a variation on other forms of fellatio. It may be difficult for some people to learn, however, due to the requirement of suppressing the natural gag reflex.

THE GIFT OF GAG

Thank goodness for your gag reflex. It prevents you from choking and besides, guys like to hear you gag. In fact, it makes them think they're so big that you just can't take them all in. Nothing like stroking the ego and the penis at the same time . . .

That being said, you don't have to like to gag, or even want to, and if you're one of those people who'd rather be gag-free, practice every morning and night while brushing your teeth. Move the toothbrush farther back on your tongue each time your brush, and over time this will help you relax. Then you can try out your newfound skills on his happy member.

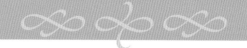

THE QUICKIE

For performing fellatio, the quickie is almost a no-brainer. In artistic terms, think of it as a sketch before your painting. As a pre-going-to-work ritual, we can't recommend it enough to start the day off right. For men, the excitement of a good blow job can almost guarantee a quick finish, so try to constantly be aware of opportunities.

However, don't get preoccupied with the climax; a few licks or strokes can be plenty of motivation for a hot interlude *later*. Got a couple minutes in an empty elevator? Drop his pants and give him twenty licks! Does she have an easily raised dress or skirt on? Reach your hand down and massage her vulva when no one's looking. Find yourselves in a secluded parking garage? Recline your seat and give 69 a try.

TANTALIZING TIPS

❧ To make him come quickly, have him assist you by stroking himself as you use your mouth to lick the head of his penis, letting your saliva run down to help lubricate his shaft.

❧ BDSM play is the perfect time to work on those communication skills. Blindfolds have a magical capability to reduce inhibitions in both partners, so take this time to seductively speak to each other. Tell your restrained subject exactly what you're going to do and order him or her to acknowledge your seductive powers.

BONDAGE LITE

Spice up going down with some light bondage and sensory play. BDSM (bondage, domination, submission, and masochism) can be an exciting way to amplify sensations during any type of sexual situation. Blindfolding and depriving your lover of sight, for example, awakens other senses—especially touch—as you slowly tease and tantalize your subject's body. It's wonderful to focus on neglected areas of the body and never let on when you'll finally attend to the genitals.

To get into the mood, consider purchasing a few well-chosen accoutrements. How about a hot latex or leather outfit befitting the task at hand? Adding a pair of hand and/or ankle cuffs can also heighten the erotic tension as the dominant position holder draws out the experience into a torture chamber of pleasure. Use light breaths and a little imagination to make your adventure more mysterious (we like to add ice or warm chocolate) and keep things away from the vagina or penis until the tension is sufficiently high.

Many items you already have make great tools for BDSM play. A spatula for light spanking, scarves for blindfolding and tying your partner to the bedposts, and a bucket of ice make ideal (and affordable) tools for torture.

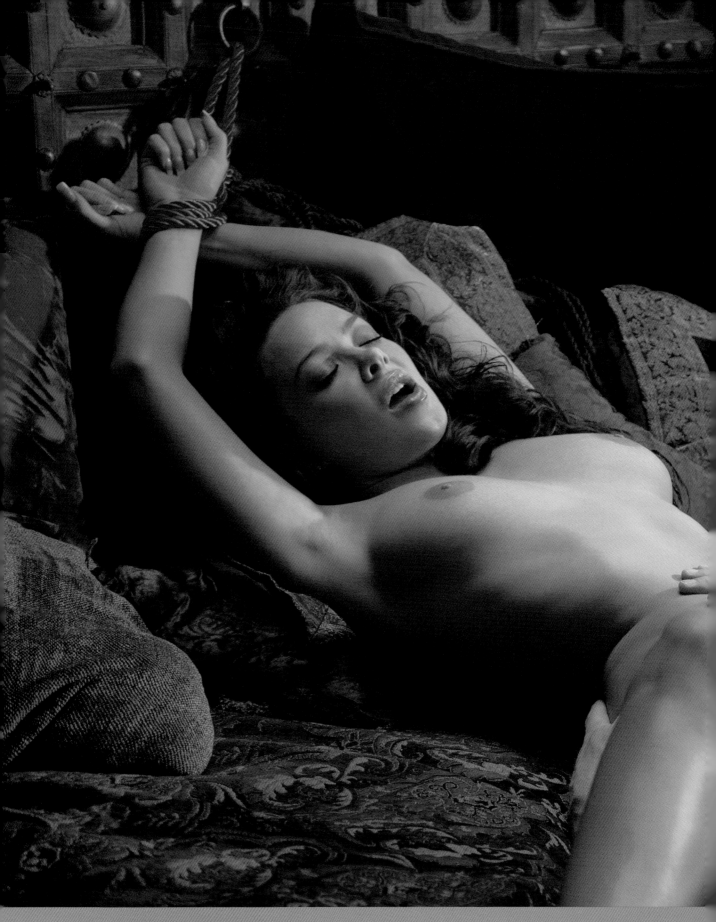

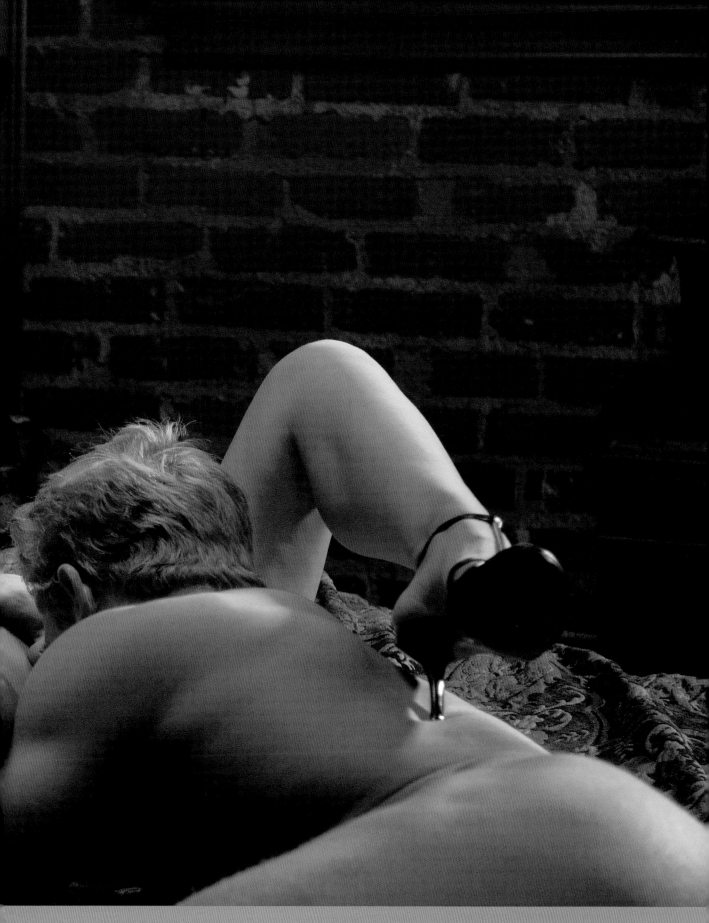

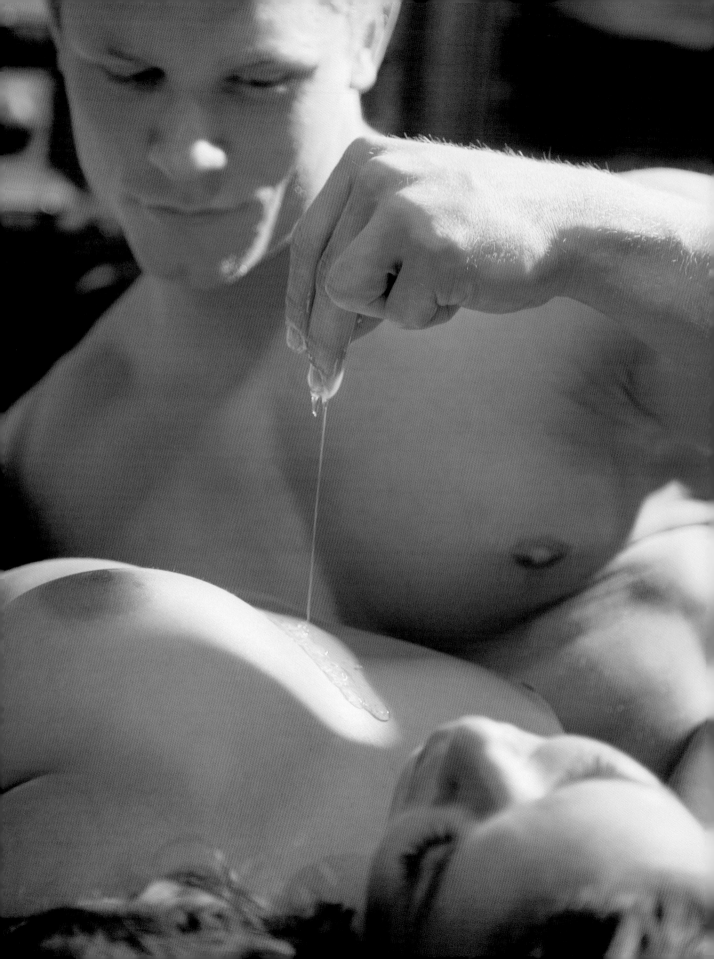

9

THE HANDS OF AN ARTIST:

Sensual Massage

"He moved his lips about her ears and neck as though in thirsting search for an erogenous zone. A waste of time, he knew from experience. Erogenous zones are either everywhere or nowhere."

—JOSEPH HELLER
AUTHOR OF *CATCH-22*

GENITAL MASSAGE can heighten arousal states for amazing results when going down. From the giver's perspective, massage is an irresistible way to get in touch with every curve and crevice of your lover's body; for the recipient, a good massage can almost be other worldly, taking your tensions away and refocusing your energies positively and sexually. If you don't already own one, you can't make a better investment than a good quality massage table, which can be found for about 200 to 250 U.S. dollars in regular department stores.

Many people think of sensual or erotic massage as the ten-minute back rub you give your partner as a prelude to doing the nasty. Not true. Sensual massage can be a fulfilling sexual experience in and of itself. Imagine: after stroking your lover into a deep state of bliss, you can bring him or her to an earthshaking orgasm—with your fingers and/or mouth.

Everyone should try sensual massage: longtime married couples, live-in lovers seeking spice for their comfortable relationships, new couples hoping to learn more about one another, same-sex, heterosexual or multipartner couples, tawdry affairs, vacation flings or anyone looking to connect with their partner in a new, exciting way. As sensual massage is less threatening than "traditional" forms of intercourse, it can be a great way to safely experiment with new ideas, partners or forms of sexual identification.

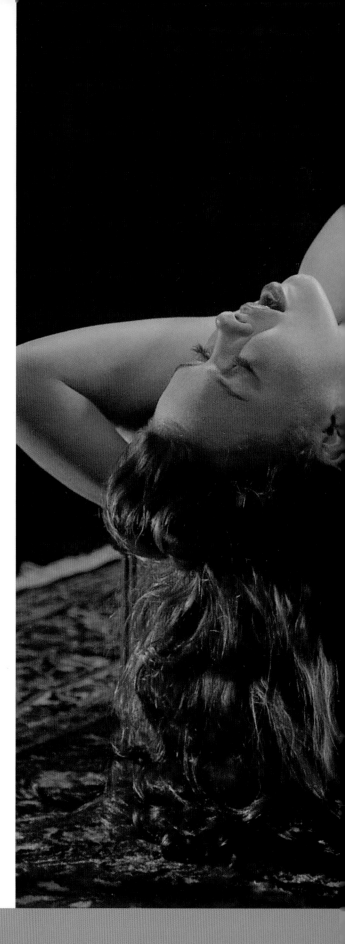

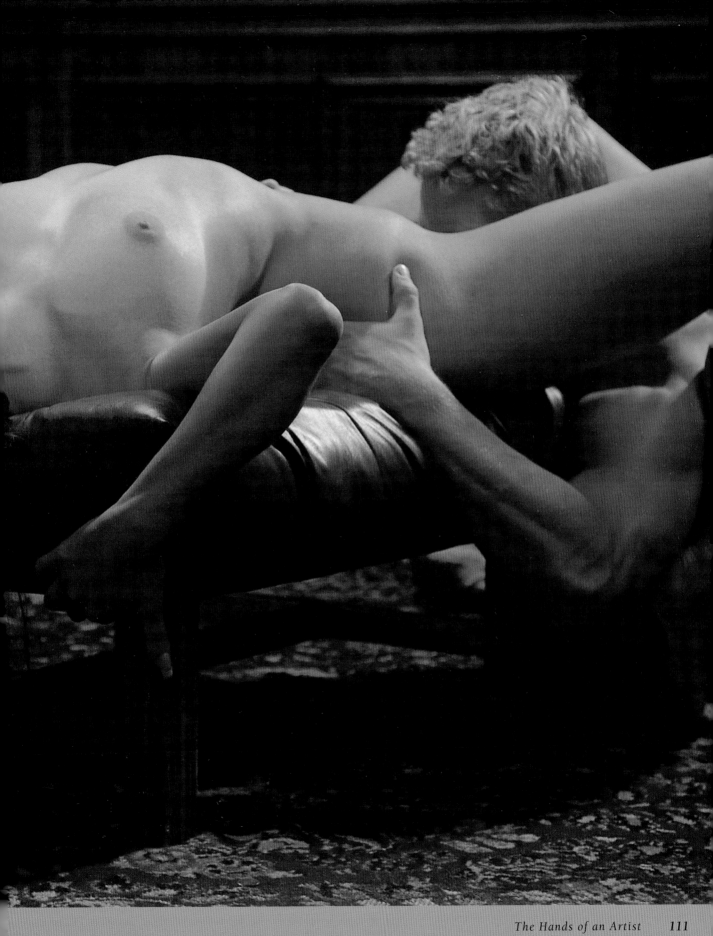

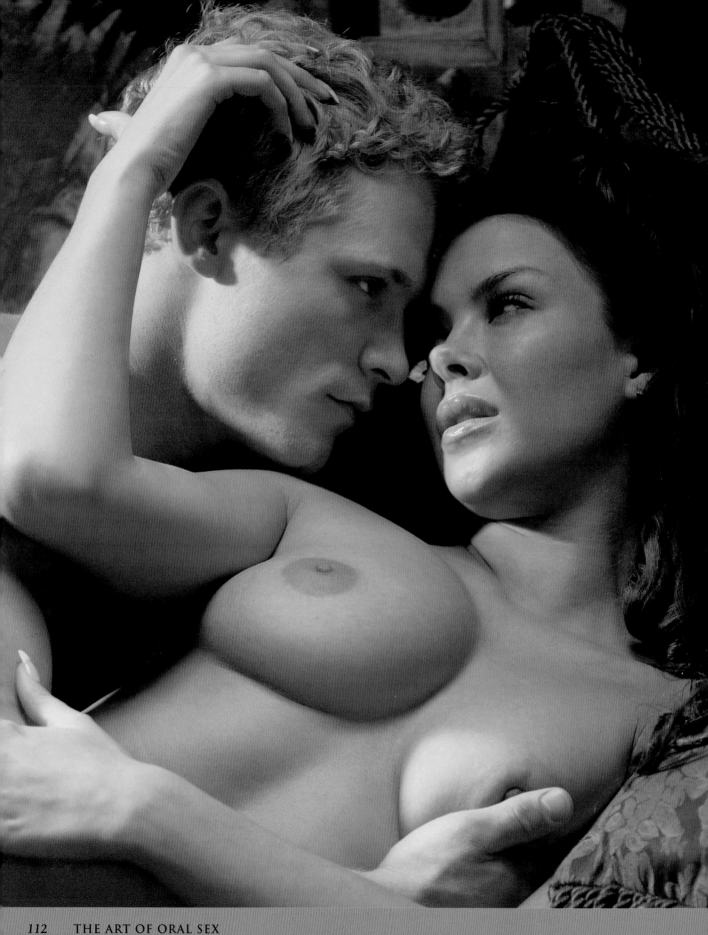

SET THE MOOD

The first step to sensual massage is creating an appealing atmosphere, one that caters to all five senses. Here are some important factors to consider when creating the right mood.

CREATE QUIET

Lock the door, turn off the phone's ringer and make sure you aren't disturbed for a few hours. Don't forget to turn off your cell phone, pager, and computer.

APPEAL TO TOUCH

If you have a massage table, use it. If, like most of us, you do not, then use the bed. Change the sheets, fluff the pillows, and fold down the covers in an appealing way. You might want to place a clean white sheet over your bedding to protect it from the oils and other liquids used in sensual massage. Provide your partner with a satin, silk, or terry-cloth robe to wear before and after the massage; choose something comfortable and pleasing to the touch.

APPEAL TO SIGHT

Turn off any lamps or overhead lighting and illuminate the room with scented candles or oil-burning lamps. Place a bowl of fresh fruit or flowers on the night stand. Hide anything unsightly, such as laundry or dirty dishes.

APPEAL TO SMELL

Burn some sensual or aromatic incense, such as lavender, ylang ylang, sandalwood or nag champa. But make sure your partner isn't sensitive to certain smells—some people react to incense with headaches, nausea, or worse.

APPEAL TO TASTE

Have a pitcher filled with cold water nearby. You might also consider a bowl of strawberries, a few pieces of rich chocolate, or some other small finger food you know your partner loves. If you and your partner drink alcohol, uncork a bottle of good champagne—but don't get too intoxicated.

APPEAL TO SOUND

Fill the room with sensual music. If you don't have a multi-CD changer, make sure to select "repeat" on your CD player. The last thing you want to do is stop the massage to change the CD.

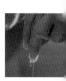

TANTALIZING TIP

Turn those cell phones, laptops, and other pesky devices OFF. It may sound obvious, but try to eliminate as many distractions as possible when setting your canvas for a perfect evening. The perfect blow job doesn't need to be interrupted by an annoying ring tone, nor does her orgasmic crescendo deserve an interruption to check that latest e-mail!

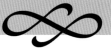

GET READY, GET SET

Start with a shower. If you and your partner are already sexual with one another, take your shower together. If not, shower before he or she arrives, and encourage him or her to do the same. Remember to have clean towels and luxurious bath products available; you want sensuality to be the theme for the night. Clip your fingernails. This cannot be stressed enough.

Having a couple of towels nearby would be smart. When lying face up, many are more comfortable with a rolled towel underneath their knees or ankles. Likewise, when face down, many people prefer to rest their head on a towel or pillow.

Other than a quiet, appealing space, you don't need many props for a satisfying sensual massage. You might want feathers, toys, or other tantalizing objects nearby, but all you really need is a good bottle or two of flavored massage oil and some lubricant to be used when massaging their genitals. Use oil-based, water-based, or silicone-based lubricants on men; but to avoid vaginal infections, only use water-based lubricants on women.

COMMUNICATION & CONNECTIVITY

Before embarking on your sensual massage, it's vital to establish exactly what your partner should expect. If he or she has never had a sensual massage, it might be good to let your subject know the differences between, say, a Swedish massage and genital stroking. Encourage frank conversation and figure out likes and dislikes; does she prefer classical music as opposed to electronic? Is he allergic to certain oils or lubricants? Is there an off-limits area, such as the anus, or is he ticklish under his balls? Try to be honest and avoid surprises.

Establish connectivity by following your

DID YOU KNOW?

Certain lubricants can irritate. When giving your lover an erotic massage, be careful to use oils that are specifically created for erotic massage (they will say so on the label) or glycerin-free personal lubricants.

"*The body is your temple. Keep it pure and clean for the soul to reside in.*"

—B.K.S. IYENGAR

YOGA INSTRUCTOR AND AUTHOR OF *LIGHT ON YOGA*

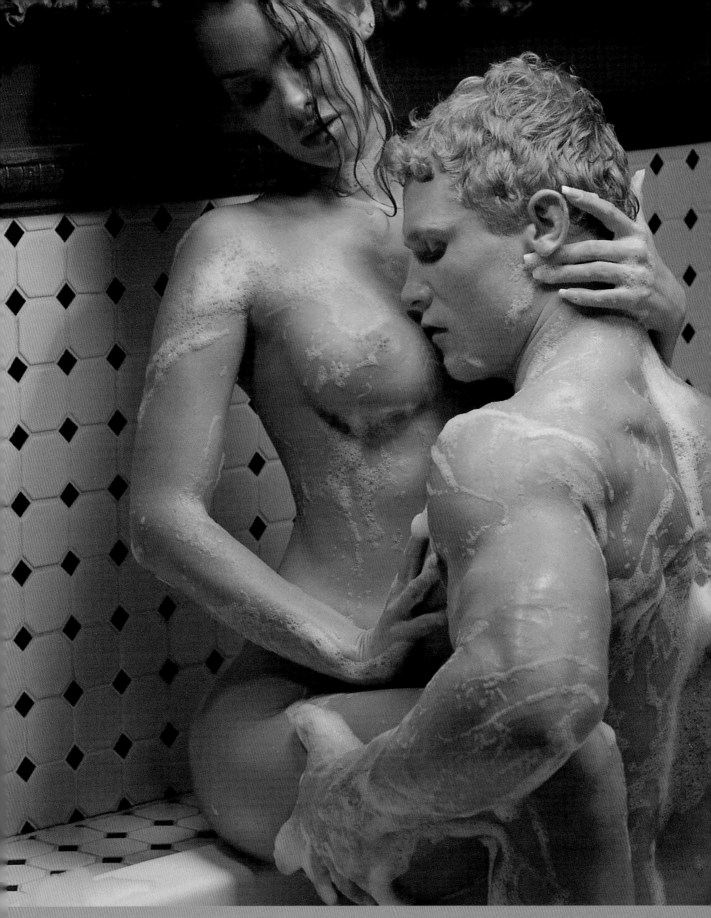

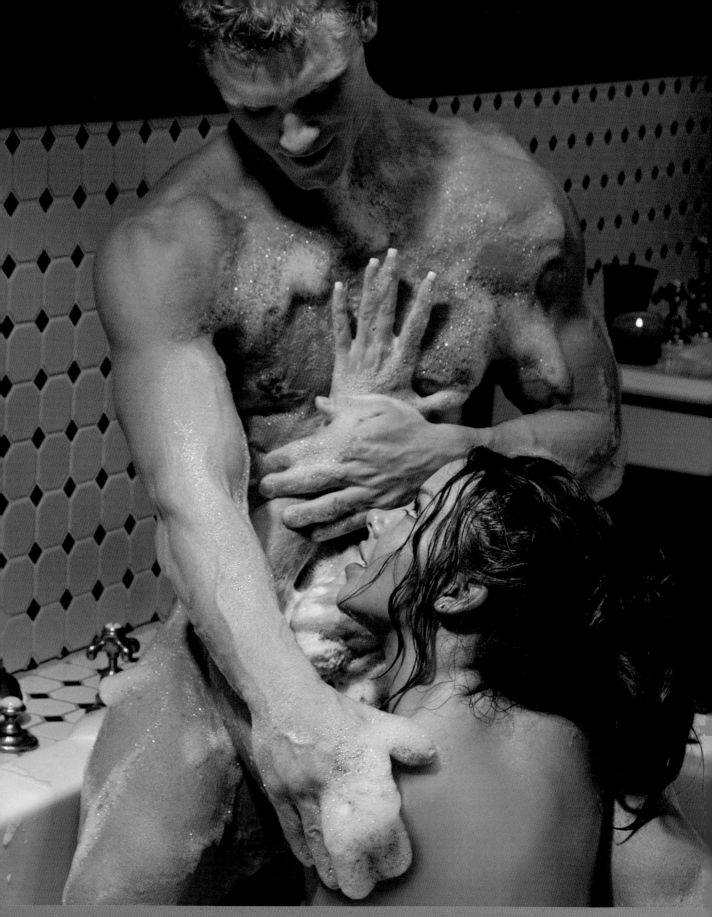

instincts. If you've been together awhile, you should have at least an inkling of what turns your partner on or how to get her relaxed. Sometime we, for example, meditate together prior to sensual massage, establishing eye contact for prolonged periods and gradually bonding as our breaths become in sync. We then lightly caress each other and kiss while maintaining focused gazes. Once you feel totally connected, you can then proceed to the massage table or well-prepared couch or bed.

RELAXATION

No matter what style of massage, relaxing your subject should be the impetus for going forward. Begin by lightly running your fingers (first the tips, then the pads) the entire length of your partner's body, bringing your face close enough so that she can feel your breath against her flesh. Progress to your palms, so that your whole hand comes into contact with your partner's body as you slowly stroke, focusing your energies around the buttocks and inner thighs in preparation for what's to come.

MASSAGING THE BODY

Cup your hand and pour approximately two tablespoons of massage oil into it, warming it sufficiently in your hands before applying it to your partner's body. We like to use massage candles, which when heated melt into warm massage oil that can be poured into use. With long, steady strokes, work the oil into your partner's body, developing a steady rhythm that continues throughout the rest of the massage. Don't be hesitant to use lots of oil and let things get slippery (just be sure to lay a towel down if you don't want to stain the sheets).

Once things get going in earnest, use both hands to cover the length of the body, paying slightly more attention to the genital areas—not the genitals themselves—and not forgetting to stop by the feet and hands along the way. Try to tease the erogenous zones as you go, watching for telltale signs (hips raising, gentle moans, slight movements when you hit a particular area of interest, etc.) that signal you to proceed further toward sensual pleasure. At this point, maybe just *brush* the genitals and see what happens. The point is to build sexual energy and maximize orgasm *later*. Once you both feel comfortable enough to begin genital stimulation, establish eye contact as you slide your hands into position.

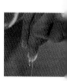

HANDS-FREE MASSAGE

Sensual massage involves more than just the hands. Use your mouth and tongue to tingle and stimulate as you advance through your partner's genitals and body. As you part her lips with your fingers, for example, run your tongue lightly inside her opening, carefully avoiding the clitoris. Or try taking her toes into your mouth one by one, using your mouth's pressure and suction to tug and tease them.

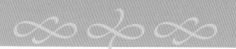

MASSAGING THE FEMALE GENITALS

As you reach your female lover's genital area, it's best to start broadly, then move down to specific areas, such as the vulva, clitoris, and G-spot, before finally diving into clitoris *and* G-spot stimulation.

Before penetrating the vagina, however, keep in mind that your female subject should be suitably aroused/lubricated, and if you're going to use a vibrator to assist in your endeavor, keep it nearby to avoid awkward pauses in your journey south.

STIMULATING HER CLITORIS

Building on your communication, try to find out as you go what feels best to her. Circling softly with your well-lubricated finger (and we can't emphasize enough the word "gently") is a good way to start, progressing as you receive feedback either through direct verbal response or body language. Think of your massage as a voyage of discovery for the both of you and focus on those destinations that steer her vessel toward the buried treasure called orgasm. Experiment, for example, by running your finger just inside her vaginal walls as you circle her clitoris; some vaginas will literally suck your finger inside them!

THE G (WHIZ) SPOT

Though not everyone in the scientific community is convinced the mythical G-spot exists, we can vouch from personal experience that it does—for us.

Located just inside the inner vaginal wall, this area—marked by a spongy, sometimes bumpy texture—can lead to mind-blowing orgasms, including those in which the female ejaculates a clear fluid similar to urine (they both exit the urethra). To put her mind at ease with regard to urinating,

TANTALIZING TIP

Raise her stimulation level and give a "butterfly massage" to her love box. From the top of the vagina, with your forefinger and ring finger in a V-shape, place them on the outside of her inner labia and gently tug upwards. There are a tremendous amount of nerve endings in many women in the labia, so experiment to see if you can find her outer inner orgasm.

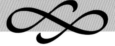

make sure she visits the restroom prior to G-spot exploration. A well-placed towel might further ease her mind and allow her to relax.

The best way to massage the G-spot is to insert one or two well-lubricated fingers into the vagina in a "come hither"-like position, then slowly move them back and forth gently, pressing slightly with the pads of your fingers. You should feel the vagina change shape, possibly swelling around your fingers as her arousal state rises. Vary your stroke pressure and speed to focus on constant pleasure, rather than orgasm. Remember, this is a massage; giving her an orgasm should be secondary to touching her with love and sincerity.

Again, keep in constant communication with your partner, either verbally or nonverbally. Watch her body for signs of pleasure or disaffection. Use varying strokes, if necessary. Above all, don't expect her to have an orgasm—just expect her to have a good time and feel good.

MALE GENITAL MASSAGE

Think of massaging the male genitals as a game of cat and mouse. You want to eat the mouse, surely, but isn't it fun to play with it before the meal? The key is to vary your speeds, stroke areas, and rhythm in order to prevent him from ejaculating, but to also give him methodical pleasure.

Ask your partner to help you monitor his pleasure levels with verbal or body language; have him moan a little louder, reach down to stop or slow you if he's getting too close, or raise his hand to let you know the peak is perilously close. Bringing him to the edge and back will reward you both with an unbelievably intense orgasm.

Although delaying his ejaculation during the course of the massage maximizes your lover's pleasure, most men enjoy finishing the massage with one, either with sex or continued massage. But be warned: ejaculation can leave men too fatigued to enjoy the rest of the evening or to do a good job massaging their partner. Partners who are reciprocating massage should therefore always have the woman receive her massage first.

Begin by applying some lubricant (*not* massage oil) to the palm of your hands and rubbing it gently into the penis and testicles. Use whatever strokes work for you and your partner, or try some new strokes. It's usually best to vary strokes at the beginning, then settle on one or two as the massage nears completion.

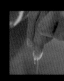

Ask your partner to help you monitor his *pleasure levels with verbal or body language; have him moan a little louder, reach down to stop or slow you if he's getting too close, or raise his hand to let you know the peak is perilously close.*

AROMATHERAPY

Aromatherapy is the art and science of using essential oils in health and beauty treatments. We use them to enhance our romantic mood, and to aid in therapeutic and erotic bathing. We love choosing massage oils rich in essential oils, specifically rose, lavender, patchouli, sandalwood, jasmine, sage, neroli, and orange for erotic massage.

WHAT ARE ESSENTIAL OILS?

Essential oils are the concentrated essence or "spirit" of plants—in other words, the natural chemical compounds which make every botanical distinctive. A specific "personality" is possessed by each plant essence: a unique scent and special properties that can be used to promote a range of therapeutic and sensual effects in humans. Essential oils have the power to heal and can be used to promote physical, mental, emotional, and spiritual well-being.

Essential oils are sensitive to light, heat, and air. Therefore, they should be stored in airtight, dark, glass containers and kept at cool temperatures. They are widely used throughout Europe, and gaining in popularity in the United States as natural remedies for a wide range of ailments such as colds, fatigue, stress, and skin rashes.

HOW TO USE ESSENTIAL OILS

The benefits of essential oils are best derived by mixing the oils with another medium of delivery like water, oil, cream, or lotion; then by using these blends through bathing, inhalation, massage, or by adding to diffusers and aromatherapy lamps. Essential oils should be used only by the drop, and like any medicine, they must be kept out of the reach of children.

In most cases, undiluted essences should not be used directly on the skin; they may cause irritation. Always dilute essential oils in a "carrier" base such as almond or other vegetable oil, before applying to the body.

Depending on the remedy, you can use an essential oil alone, or mix a few or several together in a synergistic blend. Specific oils blended together can enhance the power of the oils, amplify their energy, and deliver a more complex remedy than each of them used individually.

EFFECTS OF ESSENTIAL OILS

The molecules of essential oils are absorbed by the body through inhalation or when applied to the skin. Their therapeutic properties vary according to the specific oil or blend used. Essential oils can be used to help heal a physical problem, to alter a psychological or emotional mood, to cleanse toxins in the air, to evoke romance, or to facilitate meditative

DID YOU KNOW?

Massage has been practiced for thousands of years by virtually every culture across the globe, the oldest known written references being in China around 3000 BC. Erotic massage is thought to have first developed in India in about 2500 BC, and then spread throughout Egypt and the Greek and Roman empires.

or spiritual states. Since ancient times they have been the core ingredients in the finest perfumes, sensual oils, and lotions. Botanicals assist the body's own natural healing process. If you are unfamiliar regarding the therapeutic use of essential oils, seek out a qualified professional aromatherapist.

METHODS FOR ESSENTIAL OILS USE

Your choices are many and varied; however when preparing for the art of going down, the bath and massage are good choices.

- **Bath**: Mix three to nine drops of essential oil into a cup of sea salt or Epsom salt and add to warm bath water. Relax in bath for twenty minutes.

- **Inhalation**: Place two to three drops of essential oil on a tissue or cotton ball and inhale.

- **Massage**: Add three to ten drops of essential oil per ounce of natural, unscented massage or body oil. Massage sparingly over body. Allow oil to penetrate for two to four hours before showering or bathing.

- **Compresses**: Add three to four drops of essential oil to a basin of water. Soak a strip of gauze or cotton in the mixture. Lie down and relax with compress applied to affected area for twenty minutes. Soak and reapply the compress several times.

- **Foot baths**: Add four drops of essential oil to warm water in a small basin and soak your feet for ten to fifteen minutes.

- **Diffusers and lamps**: Follow manufacturer's instructions regarding the proper amount of essential oils and method.

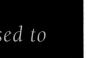

Essential oils have the power to heal and can be used to promote physical, mental, emotional, and spiritual well-being.

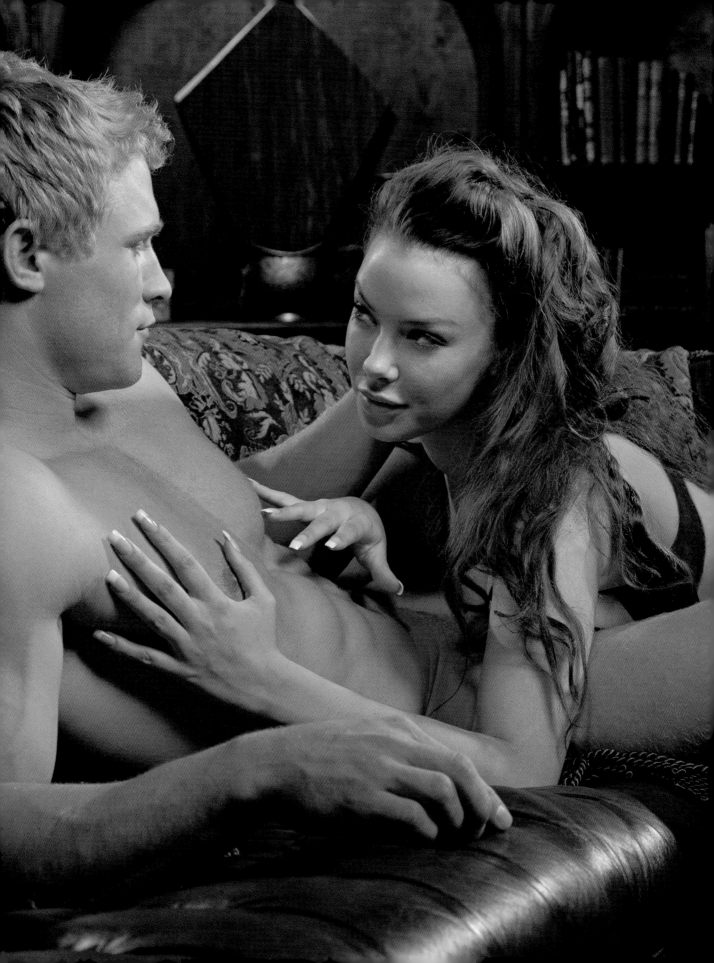

10

ADDING TANTRA TO THE SPECTRUM:

A New Approach to Oral Sex

with Deva Charu Morgan

"Tantra is the hot blood of spiritual practice. It smashes the taboo against unreasonable happiness; a thunderbolt path, swift, joyful, and fierce. There is no authentic Tantra without profound commitment, discipline, courage, and a sense of wild, foolhardy, fearless abandon."

—CHÖGYAM TRUNGPA RINPOCHE
INFLUENTIAL TEACHER OF TIBETAN BUDDHISM

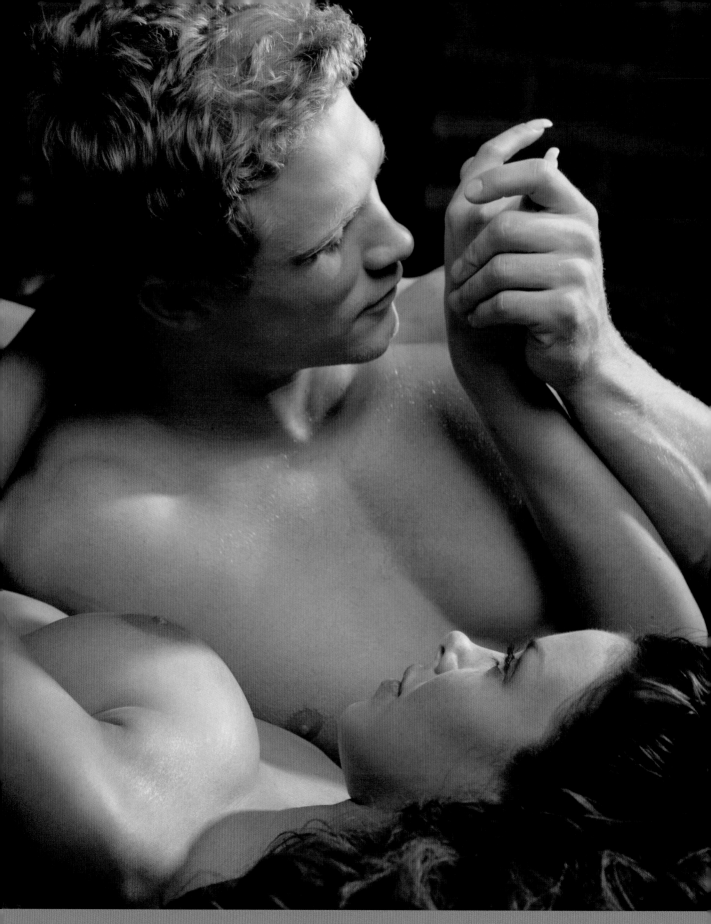

WHAT IS "TANTRA" EXACTLY? It is an ancient path of meditation where the focus is on bringing our attention back into our bodies. So often we are guided in sexual situations by our mind; ideas and patterns that our parents set for us about our sexuality; society and religious perspectives; and even by the thoughts we have ourselves about what is sexy. When we make love from this place we are limited because our mind and our thoughts know nothing of love.

Love is a sensation, it can often be triggered by the mind, but it is only by being present to this moment that we can experience love. That can be tricky to understand, but Tantra makes it simple by offering you practices to get back to what your body is feeling in any given moment. This can help you to stop paying attention to the endless meanderings and "rule making" of the mind and just enjoy what it is to be alive in this moment in this body.

For most of us, we have been making love our whole lives from our brain, so coming back to the body may feel like a challenge. That is okay. Start by imagining what it would be like if you never knew anything about sex. What would it be like to meet another human being of the opposite sex? How would you know that they are different from you? What would it be like to explore him or her and discover this new body, so different from yours? Be like a child; be like an animal. What are all of the ways in which you can explore this creature? See, hear, smell, taste, touch. This simple exercise can awaken your creativity and innocence in your lovemaking.

Let lovemaking be totally unsexy. Sexy is an idea created by society. It can be fun, but truthfully it is incredibly limited. The expanse of our sexuality is huge if you allow it to be. When you are no longer trapped by the thought of having "sexy" sex, you can give yourself the freedom to surrender to your body and your senses.

When you begin to listen to the body, lovemaking can take on a whole new texture and new levels of pleasure will be revealed to you. Trust the body, trust the senses, and you will discover your true nature: you are a multiorgasmic being with absolutely no limitations. Whoopie!

CREATE A SACRED SPACE

Creating a sacred space is such an important part of the time you set aside to be together because it can set the stage for what you will share. It is another step that conveys the message to your partner that this is important to you and that message will translate in the rest of the evening. Since often the time we have just for our relationship is limited, making the space special can help you to have the most intimate meeting with the little time you do have.

This ritual can be done on your own or together. You can take this to different levels depending on what you are comfortable with. Tantra sees making love as the greatest act of prayer, which to us simply means that it acknowledges this meeting between man and woman in love as being very powerful and holding great importance: the space will be the container for this meeting between the two of you. In the same way that when you know you are going to cuddle up and watch a movie you make some popcorn, put the pillows just so, and grab your favorite blanket, we are setting the scene for you to open up and feel sensual in an environment that you have created especially for sensuality.

THE SPACE

Choose a room or a space in your house that you would like to transform; clean it thoroughly; take out any furniture or clutter that is in the way. Create a blank slate for yourself. It would be great if this is a space that you can leave set up and come back to every time you meet. This creates what I might refer to as "an energy" in the room. If that's too airy-fairy a concept for you, think of it as a body-memory; whenever you enter this space, some part of you knows it is okay to relax and it is time to be intimate with your partner. This sensation has great power. When I walk into my own sacred space I feel very safe and my body immediately begins to open up.

THE SETUP

What makes you feel sensual? For some of us this can be as simple as making sure the bed is made; for others it will include candles, incense, flowers, or other sensual details. See if you can set aside the time to collect little objects that will help make this room special. Some ideas: a sheepskin rug (the best addition to any Tantrica's room), a vase that displays your flowers in a beautiful way, cushions, wall hangings, and art.

ESSENTIAL TOOLS

Remember that in this room the sky is the limit for your sexual exploration, so be creative in what else you will fill your room with once it is decorated. This can include oils, feathers, lubes, and toys.

(See Chapter 12 for more ideas on collecting such items.) Do not limit your choices to things you can use to please each other, but also include other items that make you feel good or remind you of something sacred about man and woman. Try crystals, different flavors of incense, a lovely yoni-shaped pillow. (Again, see Chapter 12.) Include even things as simple as a large stick you found in the yard that just felt earthy and good to you. Trust your instincts; be like a child making a fort in your parent's living room. Have fun!

MUSIC AND SOUNDS

The right music will set the mood, and for the purpose of our ceremony it is fun to collect other things that make sounds: bells, Tibetan bowls, drums, sticks you can bang together. Again, remember the energy of a child and let that guide you. Note: If this is starting to sound silly to you, I encourage you to remember that this is an experiment and it is only through experimenting that we discover new territory . . .

TANTALIZING TIP

Worship your partner's genitals. In a prayer-like pose, starting at the forehead, gently touch your lips to your partner's skin and "Oooooohhhhmmmmmm" three times slowly in a deep and loving voice. Repeat on each side of the neck, then the sternum, following with the belly button, pubic bone, and finally the vagina or penis.

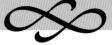

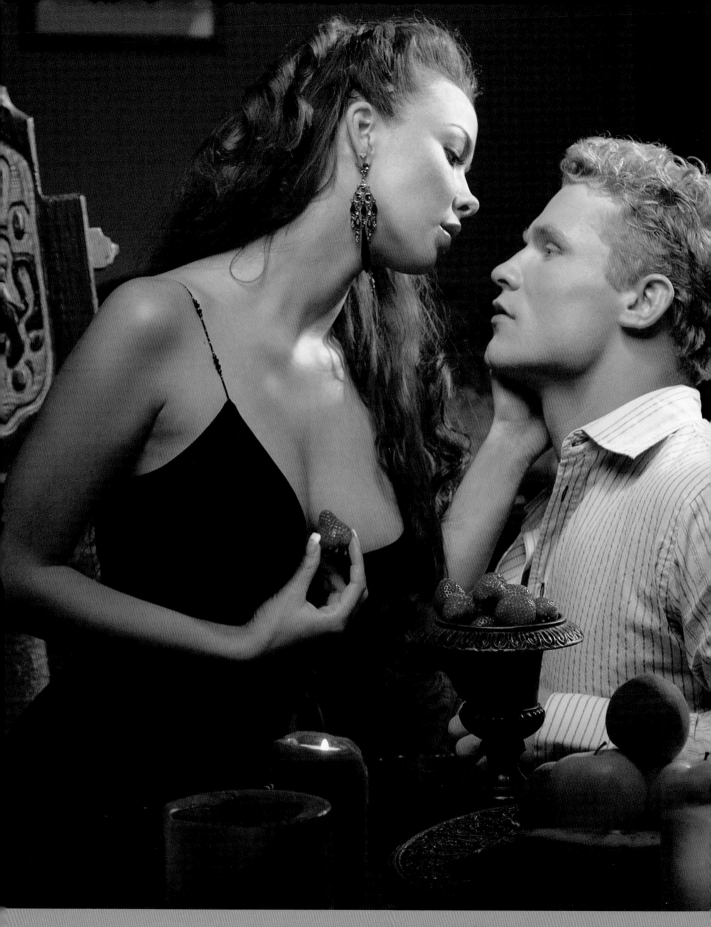

EMBRACE THE RITUAL

Now that your space is set up, you can move on to the actual ritual. Be sure to move very slowly; this is a great way to begin to step out of the pace you are moving at in your daily life and invite a new kind of relating in for you and your partner. This will set the stage for your evening and your lovemaking. As we slow down we become more aware of our surroundings, ourselves, and our partner.

As you look at this space you have created, think about what you can do to make this feel very special and sacred and what that means to you. Some people like to use sage or incense and circle the room as a "clearing" process. Perhaps you love to cook; making a meal for your love and serving it here could make this feel like home. Maybe you enjoy dancing and the space will feel full of love when you

RITUAL FOR LOVE

1. Stand across from your partner on the perimeter of what is to be your sacred space.

2. Turn to the left and walk around the space in a circle three times. These kinds of movements may feel silly, since we are not used to having an awareness of our environment; however, they are very powerful so I invite you to suspend your disbelief.

3. As you walk, think of all of the things that you and your lover would like to be free from in this space. Speak aloud, and name what you would like to "cast out." For example: "I cast out fear." "I cast out feeling inadequate." "I cast out self-consciousness." This will actually change the texture of the space. Trust me . . . nothing is too stupid to say, the sky is the limit, let go of all the things that are holding you back in this moment, holding you back from your partner.

4. You can also make sounds, use your bells or drums, or stamp your feet. Have fun!

5. After three times around, pause for a moment and notice if the space feels any different.

6. Then begin to circle in the other direction, this time "calling in" all of the things you would like to be in the room for this meeting between you and your beloved. For example: "I call in love." "I call in sensuality." "I call in playfulness." You can also use your sound-makers here.

7. Now stand still across from each other, close your eyes, take a few deep breaths, and feel the room. You may now open your eyes and step into this space you have created.

Congratulations! You now have the perfect place to explore your beloved for the first time, all over again!

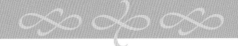

and your partner have shared a dance here. All of these are ways to make this place yours and a fertile environment for your love to grow. "Ritual for Love" on page 128 is one example of a specific tantric ritual for creating a sacred space, it is by no means the only way to do it. Have fun, be creative, and trust what feels right to you.

Remember that you can use your space for anything that feels good to do with your partner including reading, massage, and holding each other. In this case we will use it to set the stage for discovering oral sex in a whole new light.

SENSUAL MASSAGE WARM UP

Feel free to follow your heart with this one. We all have some idea about how to love up our partner using a little oil and our two hands—or other body parts! I encourage you to explore your lover's body, trust yourself, and have fun. For those who are looking for a little more guidance, try this simple exercise:

❧ Choose who will give and who will receive first.

❧ Decide how long you would like to spend on each partner. (Bear in mind that this is simply a first step for the oral exploration you are about to embark upon. A good starting point is about a half hour for each person.)

❧ The partner who will receive lays down (preferably naked) with his or her eyes closed; partner who is giving sits alongside.

❧ The massage is divided into four easy stages:

1. Sweep your hands over your lover's body slowly. Imagine you are massaging the air around their body. (Trust me, they will feel it.)

2. Softly touch this body before you in long strokes, tuning into the skin.

3. Now add pressure, connect with the muscle of this human being.

4. Finally, connect with the bones in firm loving touches.

Take a few minutes with each of these stages and when you are done, repeat them in reverse order for just a minute each; bones, muscle, skin, aura (energy around the body).

❧ When you've finished, lay beside your lover in a spoon position. Leave plenty of time for him or her to enjoy what you have given before you switch places.

TANTRIC TECHNIQUES FOR ORAL PLEASURE

Now that you and your partner are warmed-up and attuned to each other's sensuality, it's time to concentrate on other pleasures.

Take approximately five to ten minutes for each part of the following steps:

❧ The woman begins by using the man's hand. She shows how she would like to be pleasured by kissing his hand the way she would like her "yoni" (vagina) to be kissed. She should be sure to specify which part of the hand is representing the clitoris and the outer and inner labia. Her kisses and strokes can be as specific as she would like them to be

❧ The partner shows her that he has understood by doing what she has shown him.

❧ When he has finished, he may ask her, "How was that? Would you like to show me more?"

❧ The woman then demonstrates more desires to her partner—this time by using his lips to represent her "yoni." She should show anything that she would perhaps like done differently or that she would like more of, again taking special care to be specific. She may choose to use his tongue to represent the aroused clitoris.

❧ The man once again shares what he has learned by kissing her in that way on her "yoni."

❧ TIME MUST BE TAKEN WITH EACH STEP.

❧ Change roles.

❧ The man uses the woman's tongue to demonstrate how he would like to be orally loved by her. (This exercise can also be done by using one of her fingers, but in my experience this can sometimes be challenging for men who might be self-conscious about what it looks like. By using the tongue, the couple has an opportunity to enjoy a unique kiss in the process.)

❧ The woman then pleases him with the techniques he has shown her.

❧ When woman has demonstrated what he has shared with her, she will ask him the questions, "Was that to your liking? Is there anything else you would like to share with me?"

❧ The man once again demonstrates what he would like, using her finger or tongue.

❧ Once again, the woman takes her lover in her mouth and demonstrates what she has learned.

THE GOAL

Tantra should be used as a springboard; not as a destination. This is not a goal-oriented process; don't fixate on having an orgasm. In fact don't think about orgasm at all; simply enjoy the feel of your lover's tongue on your body.

When you complete the exercise above, take the time to hold one another, perhaps spooning and even sharing how it was for you. Every response is okay. Some useful starters might be: "I loved it when you . . ." or "I never knew you liked it when I . . ." or "It was weird for me too when . . ."

When it comes to defining "great" oral sex, many of us measure it on how quickly or how forcefully we are able to orgasm. But Tantra asks, "What would happen if you stayed totally present to your body, to every sensation? What experiences might we be overlooking by simply going for what we know will work?" As a couple, our most orgasmic experiences have emerged from simply feeling each other's lips on the labia or frenulum, the teeth gently tugging at the skin around the vulva and the breath on the area as the lips are held open . . .

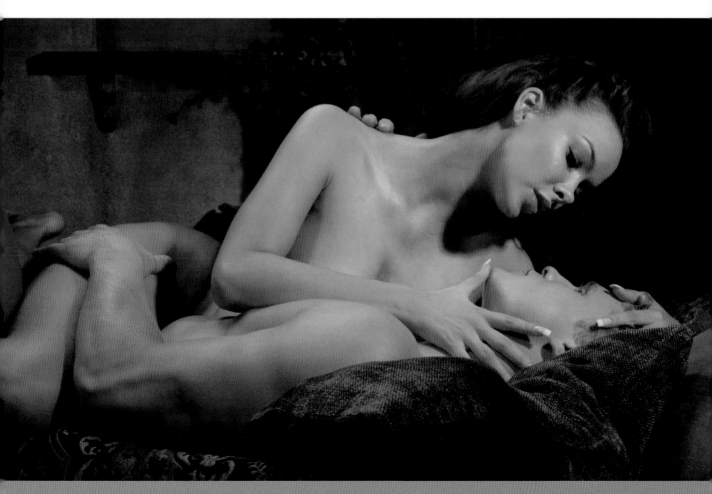

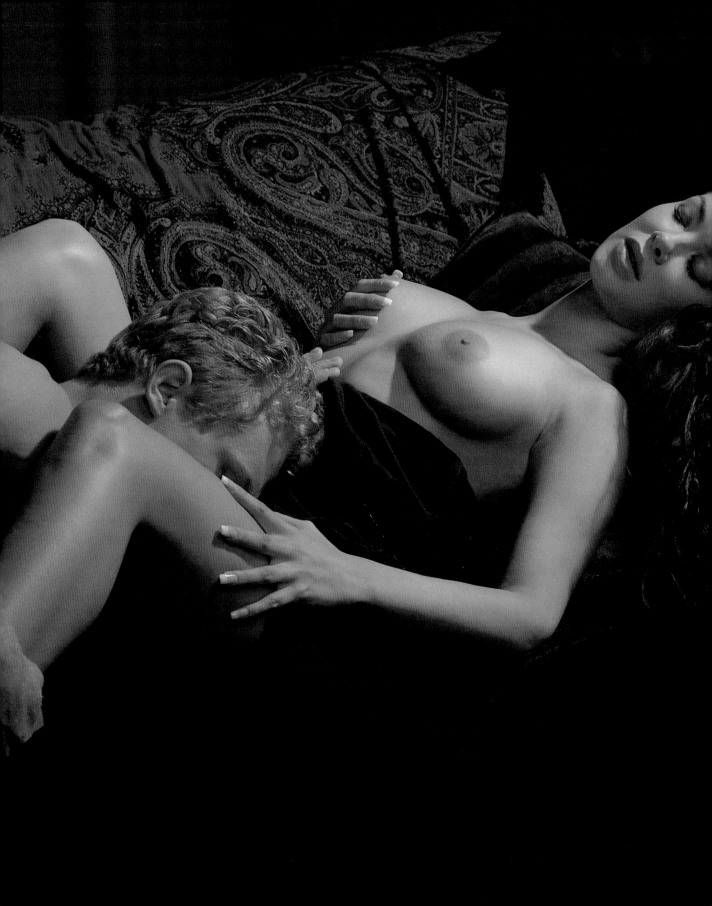

LOVING A WOMAN THE TANTRIC WAY

Taking a moment to connect with your deep love for woman, and for this woman before you, can be the most important part of the process. What a woman responds to, more than any technique, is your reverence for her. Experiment with ways to make your every move an offering of love to her.

Women are not genitally centered the way men are; they awaken sexually with stimulation of every part of their body. This means that she will respond more if you pay attention to the *whole* of her body rather than just her vagina. Here are a few things to try to awaken her sensual feelings.

- Love her thighs, legs, feet, belly: kneading, squeezing, soft slapping, and kisses will engage her senses.

- Love her breasts! Breasts in a book about going down? Yes, indeed. Tantric practices offer that it is in loving the breasts that the vagina truly opens.

- Breathe into her "yoni." (Play with the sensation of hot breath and cool blowing.)

DID YOU KNOW?

In Eastern reflexology, the tongue is believed to be connected to the clitoris on a woman and the head of the penis on man. Keep this in mind when using your partner's mouth to show him or her how to pleasure you!

- Caress, kiss, suck, and bite the outer and inner labia. (These lips often get ignored since they aren't considered hot spots for orgasmic response, yet bringing sensitivity to the area can ultimately create an opportunity for greater overall pleasure.)

- Talk to her "yoni." I know, it sounds funny. But just as your woman loves hearing you whisper sweet nothings into her ear, she may also love this experience as you love her vulva. Some women are afraid that it is ugly or strange "down there"—speaking to this part of her, and sharing your love might be just the thing she needs to trust that you are enjoying every minute of this.

What a woman responds to, more than any technique, is your reverence for her.

LOVING A MAN THE TANTRIC WAY

Man's penis is his kingdom, his directing force that leads him through the world. It is also the best instrument with which he can inject into his woman the loving that she craves in the depths of her soul.

Women, as you prepare to stroke and suck and love this member, really consider the man. Think of all of the ways in which he has shown up for you; all of the unique ways that he offers you his love and support. Let this act of fellatio be the most profound way of sharing your love and admiration for him, lose yourself in the act and love and love and love . . . you may be surprised to find that this can be as intensely pleasurable for you as it is for him!

Try some of these techniques to open your mind to loving him the Tantric way:

❧ Love his penis the way *you* want to; experiment with not worrying about what he likes and take your own journey. Why? First, you may discover something pleasurable that you would have missed had you simply been doing what you know he likes. Second, he will *feel* it. Whether or not it gets him hard, your man will feel you loving his penis and that is a great feeling! He may not get to feel your enthusiasm when you are concentrating on getting the stroke just so.

❧ Feel that you are drinking him in, taking his love inside of you through your mouth. (If you are going to swallow his semen, you can feel it entering you as the ultimate gift: a very real part of himself to you.)

❧ Take him deep into your throat. This may take some practice, but the gag reflex can correlate with the vagina—as the mouth produces more saliva, the "yoni" moistens with its juices! Wonderful!

❧ As you become more sensitive to his penis, you may actually begin to feel him through all the stages of his arousal. With very heightened awareness, it is even possible to feel his orgasm through your own body!

MORE TANTRIC TIPS FOR HIM *AND* HER

1. Focus on breathing through the whole arousal process.

2. When you near orgasm, take a deep breath and imagine the sensations in your genitals rising through your body to the tip of your head. As you exhale, feel them gently coming down again, like a breeze. This can help to expand the orgasmic sensation throughout your body. For men this is also the first step toward becoming multi-orgasmic.

3. The perineum is the area between the genitals and the anus on both men and women. Exploring and enjoying this part of your beloved with your fingertips and tongue as you pleasure him or her can add to the fun. This can be a very sensitive area!

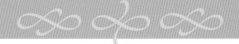

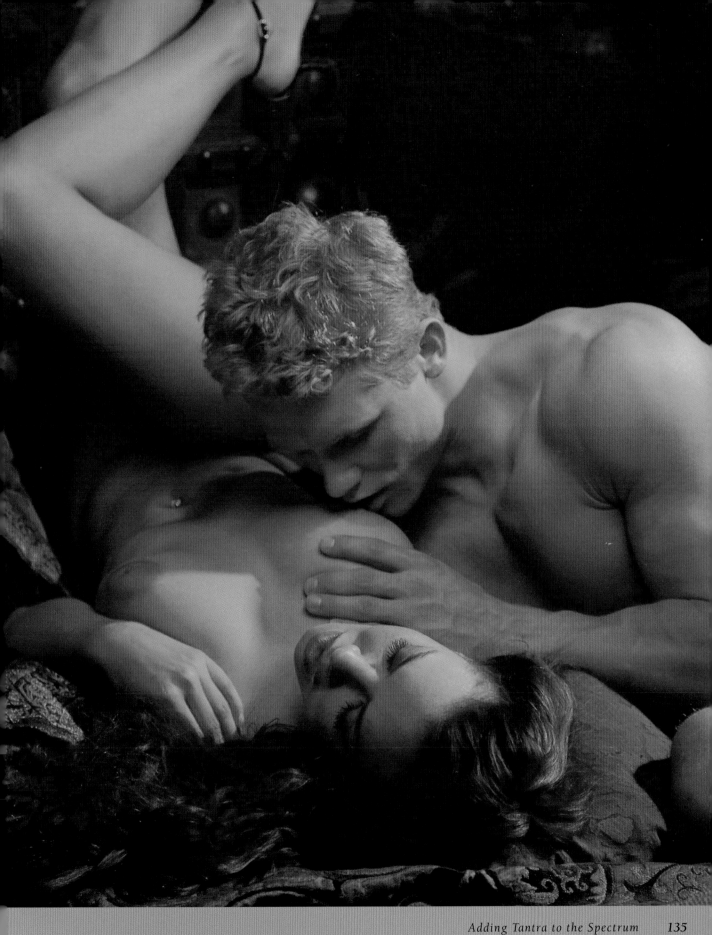

THE ALL-IMPORTANT BREASTS

As mentioned earlier, Tantra offers that it is in loving the breasts that the vagina truly opens. Loving the vagina alone, lovely as it may be, may serve to get your lover's attention, excite her, and perhaps even bring her to orgasm; however it will not *open* her. When you play with, suck on, and simply adore your woman's breasts, on a deeper level you are opening her heart. The heart is a woman's main sex organ; if her heart is open she becomes more and more available to love you totally. Very few women are even themselves aware that when you focus on the vagina or clitoris alone you are missing out on the depth of lovemaking she can offer you.

What does that mean? When you are in the presence of a woman who has deeply opened to you, you know it. This is one of man's deepest longings, to meet and love the essence and power of woman.

Why would the breasts open the vagina? Tantric theory teaches that man and woman are drawn together (beyond the animal urge to procreate) because, like magnets, they each represent a positive and negative charge. ("Negative" in this case, not meaning "bad," but simply meaning "receiving.") The penis holds the positive charge, and the vagina holds the negative one. Likewise, each of us holds both the male and female polarities inside of ourselves. This manifests as the man holding a negative charge at the chest, to balance the positive charge in his genitals, and the woman holding the positive charge in her heart or breasts, balancing her negatively charged genitals. The positive or "active" charge in

each gender is the key to opening up the genitals and awakening the "flow" in the loving that is about to begin.

A less technical way to say all of this is: suck her nipples and her vagina will be yours. By sucking her breasts you are essentially opening the flow of energy in her body, activating her negative charge (the vagina) to come to a place of yearning, pulling, longing to be filled by the positive charge of the penis. Understanding this principle can also open women up to deeper orgasms. How? Well, when a woman is opened through attention to her breasts, and the magnetic poles are ignited, she is more sensitive and has brought more awareness to her vagina in a perhaps different way than she is used to. When in this state of deepest receptivity, it can become an orgasmic experience simply to take the penis inside of her.

We should remember that when we aim directly for the clitoris in oral sex we are stimulating a "negative" pole. Clitoral orgasm before penetration can even cause the vaginal muscles to tighten and spasm, ultimately making the woman's opportunity for fully and pleasurably receiving her partner in lovemaking much less likely. When a man penetrates a woman who has just experienced the spasms of clitoral orgasm, because of the tightening of the muscles he is more likely to experience premature ejaculation. Go figure!

CLOSING THOUGHTS

Most of us understand that there is so much more to lovemaking than we have been experiencing. Simply understanding a framework of how the polarities work in the body can create an opportunity for new pleasure to come forward between you and your partner. Allow yourself to be surprised by sex. Be innocent and open-hearted. Pay attention to your body; it never lies. You may be amazed as you experiment and encounter what it is that really gets you ready for love. Often people find that the very things they counted on most to get them off are the same things that were standing in the way of the orgasmic experience that their body was guiding them towards.

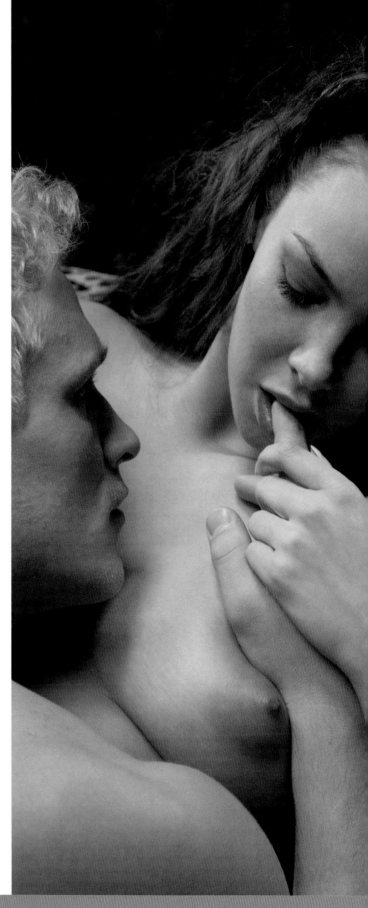

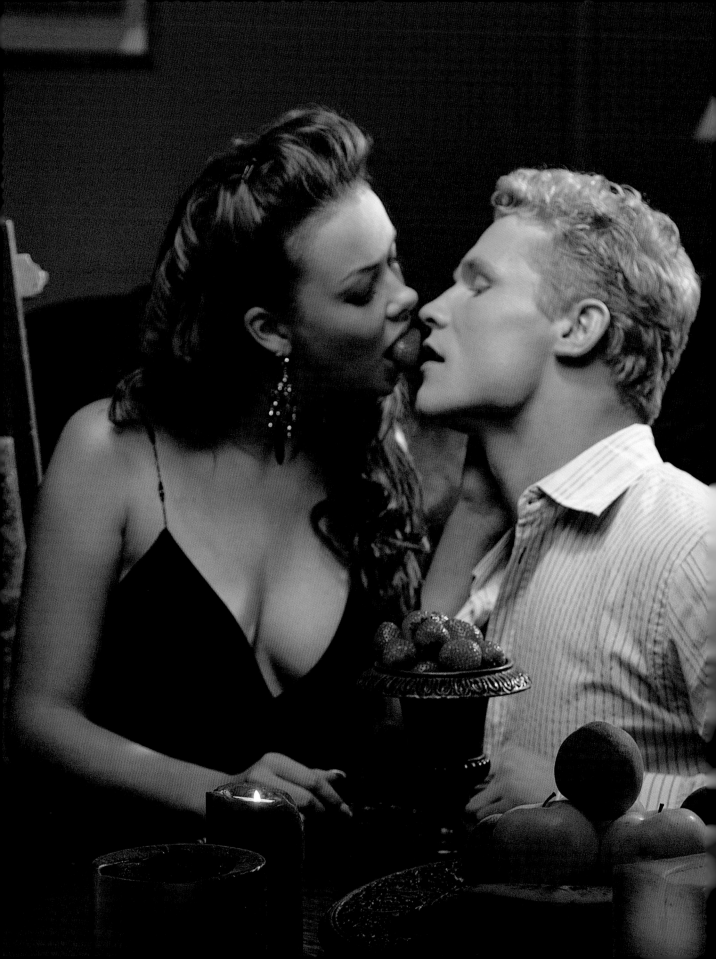

11

ARTISTIC EXPRESSION:
Oral-Erotic Stories

*"For women, the best aphrodisiacs are words.
The G-spot is in the ears. He who looks for it
below there is wasting his time."*

—ISABEL ALLENDE
AUTHOR OF *THE HOUSE OF THE SPIRITS*

A TRUE ARTIST DERIVES INSPIRATION from virtually any and all sources available to him or her: the sounds in nature, the sights in front and behind, the scents and flavors, as well as the language and words that stimulate the creative juices into action. To create art, in other words, one must be open to art. For us, erotic literature, or "erotica," is one of our most treasured pleasures and sexual inspirations. By reading the sensuous experiences— both real and imagined—of others, we ourselves can learn and be inspired to experience deeper and more fulfilling sexual interludes. The following selections contain what we consider both hot and instructive passages on journeys going down, and we invite you to share in their sensuality and allow your imaginations to paint their own vivid pictures. Once finished, we're certain your realities will far surpass these fictitious scenarios . . .

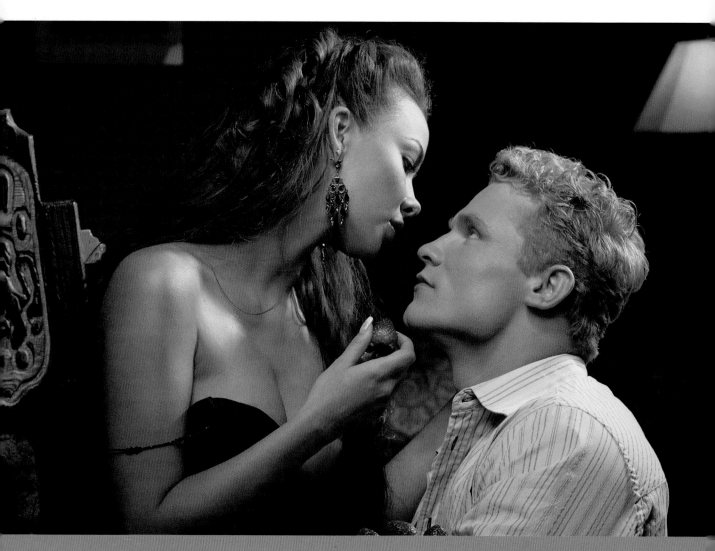

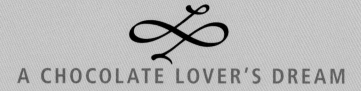

A CHOCOLATE LOVER'S DREAM

How does that saying go? *"When I was a child, I played with childhood toys . . ." Well, I have matured to a full-grown man and had put away all my childhood dreams and toys but . . . I still have a sweet tooth.*

Try as I might, I can't fight the feeling. When the urge hits me, and hits hard, there's nothing that can keep me from sweets. My tastes have matured over the years; I am not satisfied with candy I can buy at a drug store. I need sophisticated confections to fulfill my refined palette and I was craving some hot chocolate. Not even Godiva was going to satisfy this particular desire; I needed some special chocolate, and my lover Regina was just the woman to help me satisfy my cravings

MY CARNAL CONFECTION

Regina is a sexy, thick, ebony honey that drives me to distraction. I swear the Creator must have fashioned her after the Goddess Venus. She's five feet, five inches and 120 pounds of desirable Black woman. Her breasts always seem to peek out of her blouses, revealing her 36-Ds, creating that soft, pillowy cleavage that makes a grown man want to nurse again. Her chocolate brown nipples can get as hard as rocks and stick out like the tip of my little finger. I swear I could suck them for hours. Her soft round tummy and tiny waist frame the most suckable belly button you've ever seen in your life. Her hips and ass are every butt-lover's

dream—fine and heaven to hold on to when you are doing doggie style. She always amazes me at how in tune she is with her body. I swear I think she turns herself on with how sexy she is.

It's her pussy that makes a man want to fall to his knees and shed a tear, however. Hidden between those soft, sexy, brown thighs is nirvana. Within the delicate folds of her pussy are the most beautiful, crimson inner lips. They open up to one of the hottest, tightest, honey pots I've ever experienced in my life. Her slippery-sweet juices seem to flow like wine when she's aroused, and she loves to taste herself on my throbbing hard cock while I'm fucking her.

"Stop," she'll say, "let me lick all my sweet cum from that hard meat."

SHE'S MY ADDICTION

Seeing her devour my white cock like that is pleasure in ways I can't even describe. My body feels the pleasure of her soft, full lips licking and sucking, but my mind knows she's doing it to taste her own heavenly juices. I can't blame

Continued on p. 144

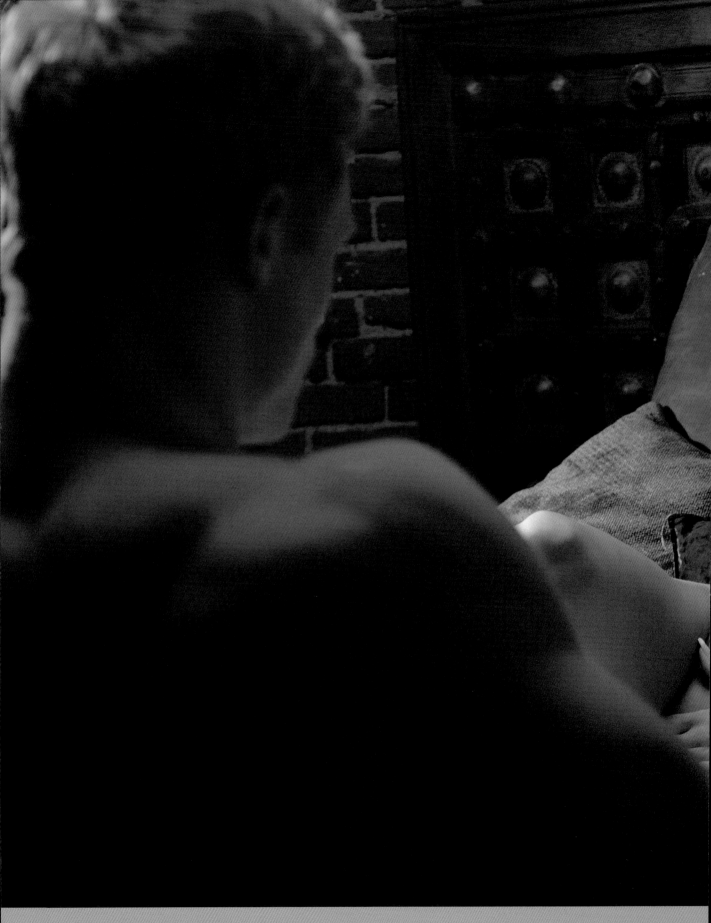

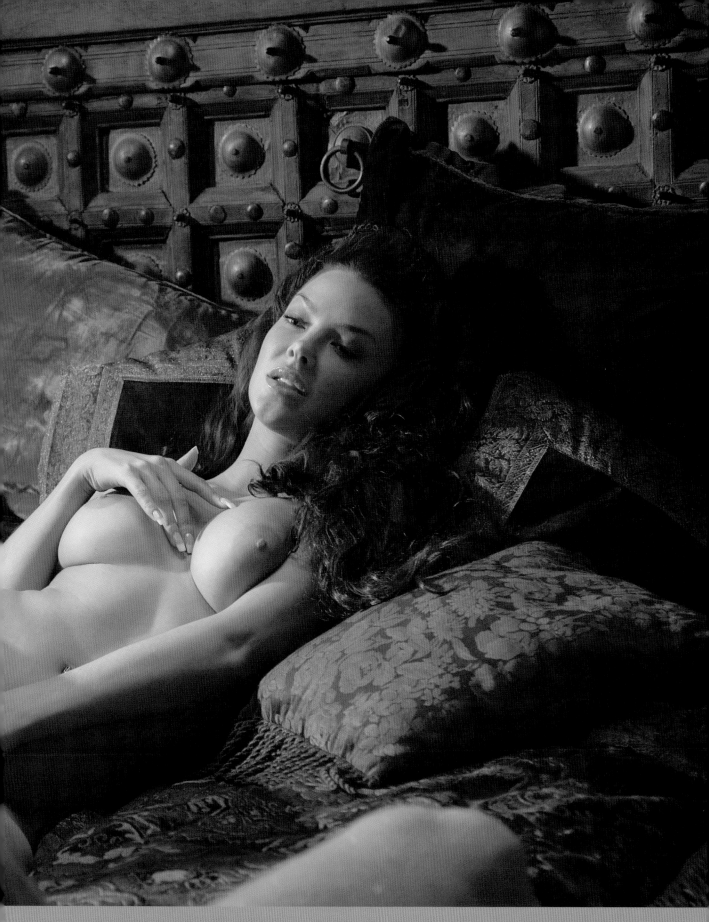

Continued from p. 141

her, I'm addicted to her taste as well, and I'd probably lose my job, house, and my car if she let me eat her out every day. I'd be so distracted with the way she moans, the way she fills my mouth with her cum, I'd probably forget to eat real food. That's how much I love going down on her sweet, black pussy.

I gave her a call on Friday night and told her that I had a very special treat in store for her. I'd gone shopping online and found the Lover's Paint Box, a set of three different types of chocolate that you can paint on your lover. I was pleasantly surprised when it arrived; it was beautifully packaged and it was sure to please Regina's aesthetic tastes and my tastes as well.

I know I'm not the only man in line for her affections, but I also know that I take my time in pleasing her and that I move to the top of the line in front of other lame guys that think they are doing her a favor by pumping her a few times and thinking that they've done something special. Me, I spend hours touching, caressing, licking, sucking, and finding ways to bring her to orgasm. I learned a long time ago to throw out everything I thought I knew about pleasing a woman every time I am with someone new. Every woman likes to be touched in a different way, every woman likes to be pleased differently, so I start from scratch and have her reveal exactly what turns her on. It takes time, but believe me it's worth it. Not only will she climax harder than she's ever come with someone who doesn't take the time to get to know her body, but she's always going to invite me back for more. Regina loves the fact that I start out slow, gentle, and tender and build up the tension. I massage every inch of

that fabulous body like I am a sculptor creating the most treasured piece of art. By the time we get to penetration, she is screaming for me to fuck her like there is no tomorrow.

AN EVENING OF SWEET SEDUCTION

She arrived Friday and she was a half hour late. Sometimes I think she does that just to keep me on edge, other times I imagine that making that body smell so good and feel so soft has to take a long time. I didn't even try to pretend to cook; I ordered Thai food and had it waiting for her when she arrived. We ate passionately, the spices and flavors stimulating us for a night that was sure to be memorable. After dinner, we made our way to my den for a cocktail. I had a bottle of Merlot breathing and she was anxious to find out what my special surprise for her was.

"You know how much I love chocolate, and you know how much your sweet honey drives me wild. Well, tonight, I thought we should combine the two. I presented her with the box I had wrapped in some left-over gold wrapping paper from some other night of seduction I'd planned for someone else, and with some ribbon from a present my mother had given me on my birthday that I had thought to save for an occasion such as this. The box was almost as beautiful as she was, sitting there in the candlelight with her shoes off and her legs under her on my sofa. She tore open the paper and her eyes danced playfully as she opened the box.

"Hmmm, I'm not sure this gift is as much for me as it is for you, sweetie," she taunted me playfully.

We laughed and I confessed that I had in fact intended to get much more pleasure from it than she would, but that it would be a close call. We opened up the jars and tasted the sweet chocolates. I loved the dark and white chocolate the best, and Regina liked the milk chocolate. When the night was over, I knew I would have my sweet tooth satisfied and a few other desires as well.

TASTING HER SWEETNESS

Regina took her ring finger and dipped it gently in the milk chocolate and stuck her finger in her mouth and started sucking it like she was sucking my cock. I got so hard so fast I felt light headed. I moved the wine glasses out of the way, knowing that things were going to get heated quickly. I started unbuttoning her blouse, and revealed a beautiful red lace bra that looked like it was straining to hold its contents. She pulled her left breast out, looked me right in the eye, and told me to put my favorite chocolate anywhere I wanted. I took the paint brush from the box and dipped it in the white first. I painted the letter R on the right side. I took the brush and dipped it in the milk chocolate next and painted the left side of her nipple with a heart. I saved the best for last, and took the dark chocolate and painted her pointed hard nipple right in the center so it looked like a chocolate chip. Picasso didn't have anything on me. She took her hands and grabbed her breast and offered it up to me. I lowered my mouth to it and tasted sweetness like I've never known. Her hard nipple, her soft brown breast, her hands pulling me to her, telling me how good my mouth felt on her, and . . . the taste of chocolate. My senses were overwhelmed.

I undressed her, she undressed me, clothes were thrown all over the floor, and we spent the next hour painting chocolate and licking it off each other's sensitive spots. She licked my sensitive nipples and had me whimpering like a baby. I put a pool of white chocolate in her belly button and licked it all out. I even painted her sexy toes with chocolate and licked and sucked them while she fingered herself to orgasm.

LOSING CONTROL

My cock was just about at critical mass when Regina reached for the milk chocolate and applied it liberally to the head of my shaft. I waited and watched. She looked up at me and licked her lips. Her mouth was like hot velvet. She licked and sucked and licked some more. She licked my nuts, which always feels so damn good. Then she swallowed my head and swirled her tongue around it in what I swear is some ancient technique she learned from a channeling a Tantric priestess. My head was spinning. I heard moaning and cursing and I realized it was me.

"Oh shit, stop," I begged her. "Please stop, I'm going to cum."

I grabbed my cock and squeezed it to keep from erupting. Once I had regained control, I grabbed her in my arms and flipped her over and lay her back on the sofa. She held her legs open and I lost my focus for a second, forgot where I was; I might have even had to think about my own name if someone questioned me at that particular second. I was in awe of her gorgeous pussy and just wanted to stare at it for a few moments.

There's something about staring at a beautiful pussy that leaves me sort of speechless. I've seen dozens in my lifetime in one form or another, but every time I'm presented with one in real life I just have to pay homage to the sweetest place on earth, the center of the universe, the place where all life comes from. It's humbling to know

Continued on p. 146

Continued from p. 145

that I am allowed such an honor as to go inside there. And the fact that it gives me so much pleasure is just icing on the cake. I could see her sweet honey glistening on her lips, letting me know she was already really aroused. Her clit was swollen and peeking out at me, calling me to it. I took my index finger and rubbed it softly, making her wiggle.

She wanted to forgo the chocolate and the licking and get straight to fucking. I would have agreed with her if it hadn't been for the fact that I never, ever, ever make love to a woman without licking her to orgasm first. It's my trademark, it's my ritual, and it works for me. No need to change game plans in the middle of the fourth quarter when I have the ball and I'm ahead.

I closed my eyes and had a moment of silent meditation. I just wanted to appreciate every second of the gift I was about to receive. With my eyes still closed, knowing her pussy like the back of my hand, I gently placed my mouth on her clit. I held it there for a few seconds, warming it with the heat of my mouth, ever so softly and gently licking it. I took my fingers and spread her lips and began to softly kiss the lips of her pussy, having them open up to me to allow me to taste the precious nectar that flowed within. I stopped for a second to use the paint brush to softly paint the outer lips of her pussy with whatever combination of chocolate remained on the brush. With my eyes wide open, I tasted her again, this time, the succulent juices of her pussy were mixed with the decadent taste of the chocolate. If Emeril knew what the hell he was doing, he would have this on the menu at his restaurant. I've got your BAM right here!

A RARE DELICACY

Regina was grinding her pussy on my face, getting me wet with her juices and I was trying to bathe in them. My mouth was alive with the sweet, salty, earthy taste of her cunt and the most delicious chocolate in the world. Well, maybe it was so delicious because it was mixed with such a rare delicacy.

Regina was chanting incoherently, "Eat me . . . lick me . . . suck me . . . fuck me . . ."

I took my fingers and inserted two inside her. I made her clit my target with my mouth and began licking her just the way she likes and fingering her. She lost control and started calling me names like a drunken sailor on a weekend pass. Her breathing was erratic and out of control. She was grinding her pussy on my mouth and she had a grip on the back of my head that the WWE would be jealous of. I felt her legs tremble and heard her muffled cries as her body tensed up.

The night was far from over, we licked and sucked and fucked each other well into the wee hours of the morning. We had chocolate for a midnight snack; we had chocolate for breakfast. I laughed when I thought about how much my trainer and my dentist would appreciate my new way to satisfy my sweet tooth.

~BY SCOTTIE LOWE

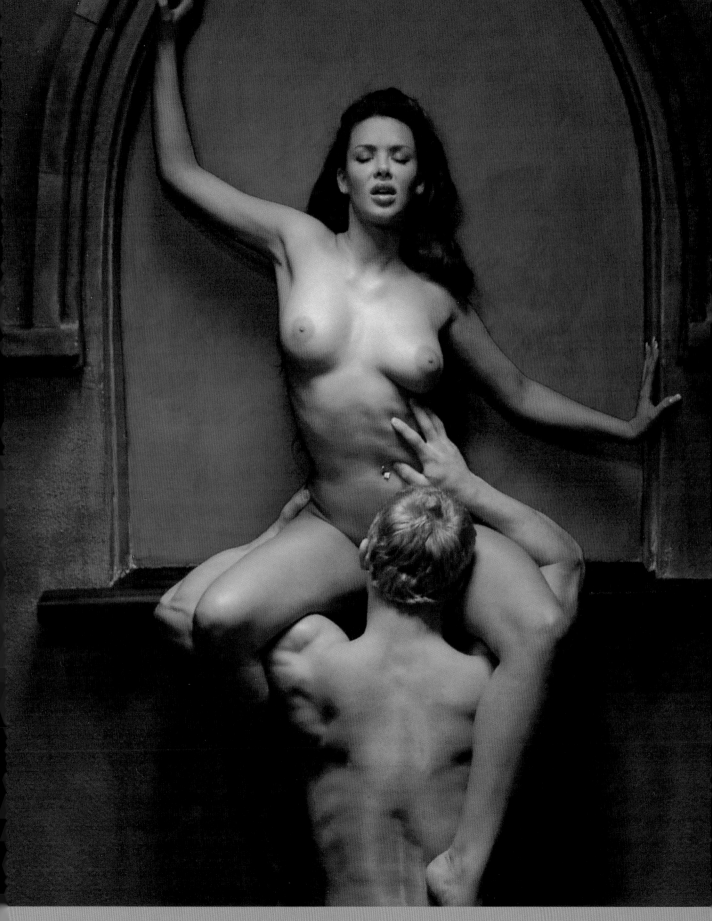

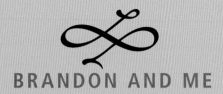

BRANDON AND ME

I met Brandon right out of a one-and-a-half-year relationship
that ended badly. A friend set us up on a blind date: drinks at a local pub
on the Plaza and "see where it went from there."

I was in my mid-twenties, and my sexual experience was limited to a handful of boyfriends who never seemed like they knew what they were doing. Even though I was inexperienced in the art of sex and sensuality, I grew very proficient at faking orgasms.

After drinks, Brandon walked me to my car, which happened to be a late model Ford pickup with a very large cab. Both tipsy, Brandon started kissing me at the truck and whispered in my ear, "There's something I'd like to do for you. Something I love to do and can do very well."

He nudged me into the truck and pulled down my slacks and panties. I became nervous and my eyes darted around the parking garage. I never, ever did anything of this nature, especially on the first date, but I was fresh out of a sexually unsatisfying relationship. Hell, I needed this.

Brandon climbed in after me and closed the door. He grinned and lowered his head, kissing my thighs before going in for the main event. Thank God I thought to shave.

I had always heard of guys who were good at oral sex, but I had never had first-hand experience with one. My experiences with men "going down" on me were roughly comparable to a cat licking milk out of bowl. It did nothing for me. However, Brandon was a bird of a different

feather. He knew exactly what to do, and he knew exactly when to do it.

I heard some voices and peered out the window to see the Plaza security guards twenty feet away from my truck, oblivious to the fact that we were even nearby. I hissed to Brandon that there were people near and we were going to get caught, but he merely grunted and kept his attention focused at the task at hand, not missing a beat. I shrugged and let him continue. It was a feeling too good to stop.

I really began to get into it, forgetting about the fact that we were in a parking garage in a very upscale entertainment district. Maybe the risk of getting caught added to the excitement. After a while, I began to feel a pull from my body's center. Sort of like the feeling you get when an airplane first takes off. I let the feeling wash over me until it felt like the world was spinning, and every nerve in my body came alive. Wave after wave of pleasure washed over me until I was left spent, my body on fire. Brandon emerged, grinning.

"I didn't know you were a squirter."

"A what?!?" I asked.

"You squirted me in the face when you climaxed."

True to his word, his face was wet. I was mortified.

I stammered profuse apologies until he silenced me with a kiss.

"Don't be. I've heard about girls who can do it, but I've never met one until now. That was amazing." I blushed. My first introduction to female orgasm, and I had no clue I was capable of such a thing, much less any other woman.

I've never been brought to orgasm in the manner that Brandon brought me to that night. It was truly a memorable experience, and he set a high bar for oral sex that no man has met since.

~BY HEATHER P.

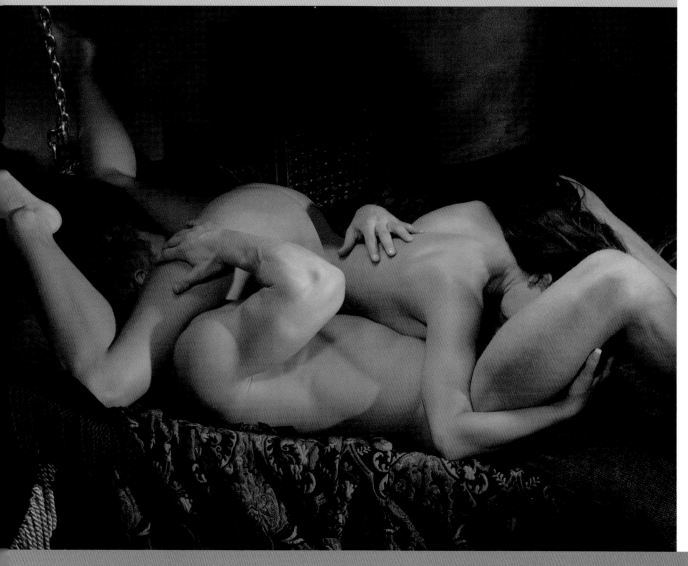

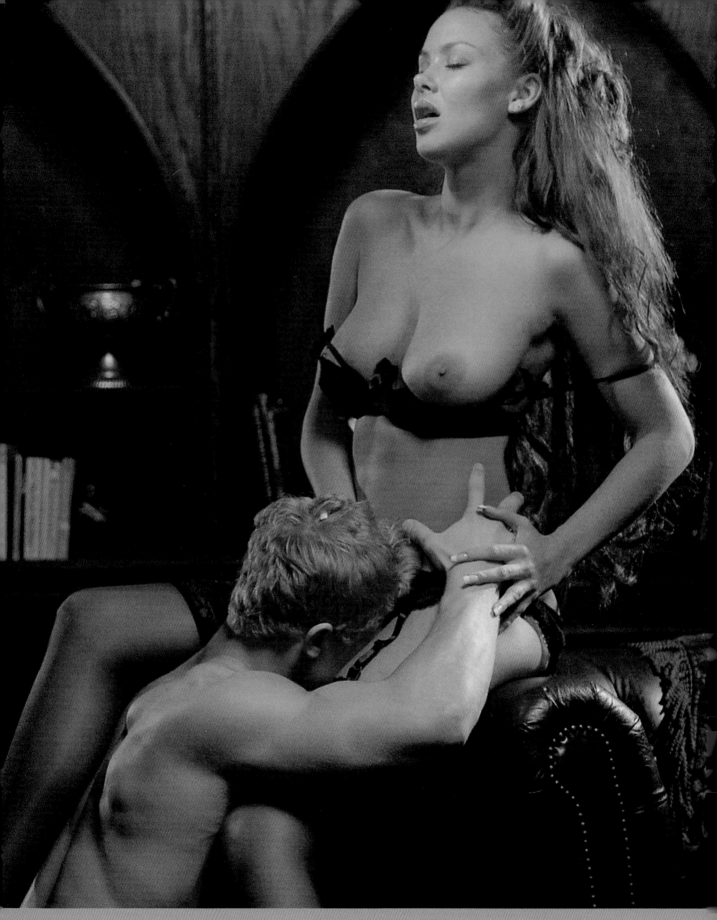

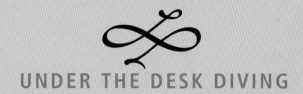

UNDER THE DESK DIVING

*. . . **I'll conclude by detailing** one of our more public exploits. One Wednesday morning, after having slept very soundly and for longer than usual, we not only awakened in the highest of spirits but with a great deal of excess energy on our hands.*

There was Caroline with her beautiful head pushed deep into the pillow, blithe eyes and laughing lips demanding kiss after kiss—kisses I eagerly dispensed. Kissing gave way to pillow and blanket fights; we were definitely of a mind to play all day. But then, it being a weekday morning, the specter of work arrived to spoil our fun. It was easy enough for me to phone my temp agencies and inform them I'd already been booked for the day; but what good was my skipping work if Caroline had to report to her job? Of course, she could phone in sick but, as undeniably wild and reckless as she was, she was also inherently responsible and disliked playing hooky, especially at this late hour when her employer would need to scramble for a replacement. On the other hand, it was such a shame to waste our riotous mood and thirst for frolic: the thought of being apart for the whole day struck us as being cruel and unusual punishment carried to its extreme.

SEIZING THE DAY

"Jobs are garbage!" I recall myself declaring as we were both stepping into the shower. "After all, here we are: two adults in the prime of life, with our juices running hot and this whole day before us, and this day doesn't belong to us! Soon you'll be at the office—later I'll probably be proofreading somewhere: it's an unpardonable waste, a sick disgrace, a joke in the worst of tastes! No more of this (I grasp and squeeze one of her soap-slickened globes) until later this evening! I might be dead of sex-starvation by then!"

The simple act of grasping Caroline's immaculate ass, on account of the degree of pleasure derived, flings me headlong into more intimate activities; soon we're intertwined on the floor of the shower with the warm water streaming over us. More diatribes against the working week and interruption of fun are indulged in; by the time we emerge from the shower we've decided that we aren't going to tolerate being deprived of each other's company, and will spend the day together regardless of the fact that she's going to work.

As I've said, it was an easy matter for me to phone my temp agencies and inform them I was unavailable for new assignments on account of already being booked. Of course, the fact that Caroline happened to work at one of

Continued on p. 152

Continued from p. 151

my agencies and that I was going to accompany her there presented a slight complication, in the event I was sighted by the director or someone else who might recognize me: I'd simply inform them I was resting up for a week-long assignment at a place known to be extremely hectic. So I made my phone calls and obtained my freedom. Thereafter, we dressed, ate breakfast, and hopped a cab to Caroline's place of employment.

A SENSUOUS SET-UP

We arrived at Caroline's workplace ahead of most of the others: it wasn't difficult for me to slip underneath her desk without being seen. As she'd said, there was a surprisingly accommodating amount of space underneath this desk—it was almost as if it had been designed with concealment of a lover in mind. Built from the floor up, there was no possibility of glancing under it except from the back and, even then, portions were still concealed from view: there were hollow spaces behind the two sets of drawers which flanked the seat of the user and if one crawled into either of these spaces one could only be discovered if someone got down on their knees and poked their head inside.

So there I was: underneath my sweetheart's desk in the reception area of a well-known and respected temp agency, as her workday progressed. She was cheerfully performing her receptionist duties—screening and redirecting calls, greeting and bantering with visitors— while thrusting her legs as far inside the desk as she could. What a view I had! She was wearing the knee-length pleated aquamarine skirt—one of my favorites—with nothing underneath and her legs were spread as far as the confines of the desk's interior would allow: how can I fully communicate the effect of this sight upon me, combined with the effect of my being hidden under her desk in a busy office? The symmetry and softness of Caroline's thighs—the moist flower between them—the sound of her voice engaged in conversing, in a very professional tone, with some new arrival! Ha, I was wildly atingle before even so much as beginning to enjoy the bounties spread before me; the simple act of running my hands up and down her calves and squeezing her thighs was good for a great deal of seeming to melt from the inside out—much of the pleasure due to the fact that I was often obliged to bite my lips and place a hand over my mouth to prevent myself from erupting with laughter. What more heady combination is there than a delicious cutie joyfully making herself accessible in a place where very few would suspect such is possible? Where others in the immediate vicinity haven't the faintest idea of what's transpiring? The juxtaposition, the contrast! The daring, the delight! The turning inside out with glee like a child hidden in a candy store and gorging himself while adults come and go! Damn! Words are unequal to the task of encompassing the amount of bliss I was under the influence of!

CLANDESTINE CLIMAXES

And when I finally (after intentionally putting it off and savoring both the sight of her and the situation) plunged my face between Caroline's thighs and flicked at her warm wetness with my tongue! How gratifying to drink of her nectar in that office environment—to tease her love-bud with the tip of my tongue while stroking her slippery canal with my fingers—to coax her towards consummation, to teasingly bring her closer and closer, only to suddenly impose a delay; and then to finally nudge her over, bring about that special inner upwelling, sigh of release. People would come and go, or the phone would ring; my dearest would be obliged to speak to them, seek to conceal her state of arousal with a flatness of vocal tone. I'd be doing my best to get her voice to tremble and crack: it was a contest we were both well aware of despite the fact that not a word had been exchanged on the subject . . . we had many laughs about it afterwards.

On a couple of occasions Caroline, on account of being face-to-face with the director or some other person of importance, was obliged to rap on the top of my head with her hand. I immediately understood that I was to temporarily halt my efforts at stimulation, and did so; then she'd nudge at me with a leg and I'd resume. And (ha! ha!) again I must mention the times I was obliged to bite my lips to stifle impending howls of laughter at the same time that I was intent upon continuing to undermine her composure and convulse her with pleasure. Nor to leave out when I later stroked myself into blissful spurtings while admiring the symmetry of her legs and slippery pink of her parted petals. I don't think I exaggerate when I insist that a man can seldom expect to enjoy as much sustained—

indeed, steadily increasing—sexual gratification as I did on that cheerful morning spent sating my hunger, contenting my imagination, and indulging the jokester in me under my adored's desk as she answered the phone, greeted visitors, and chatted with coworkers.

Yes, to hell with the Mile High Club! The club that really matters is the Under a Receptionist's Desk During Business Hours Club! Let's see how many fun-loving souls can become members of the latter!

~EXCERPT FROM "RECEPTIONIST THRILL,"
BY ROBERT SCOTT LEYSE

"*Some things* are better than sex, some things are worse, but there's nothing exactly like it."

—W. C. FIELDS
COMEDIAN AND ACTOR

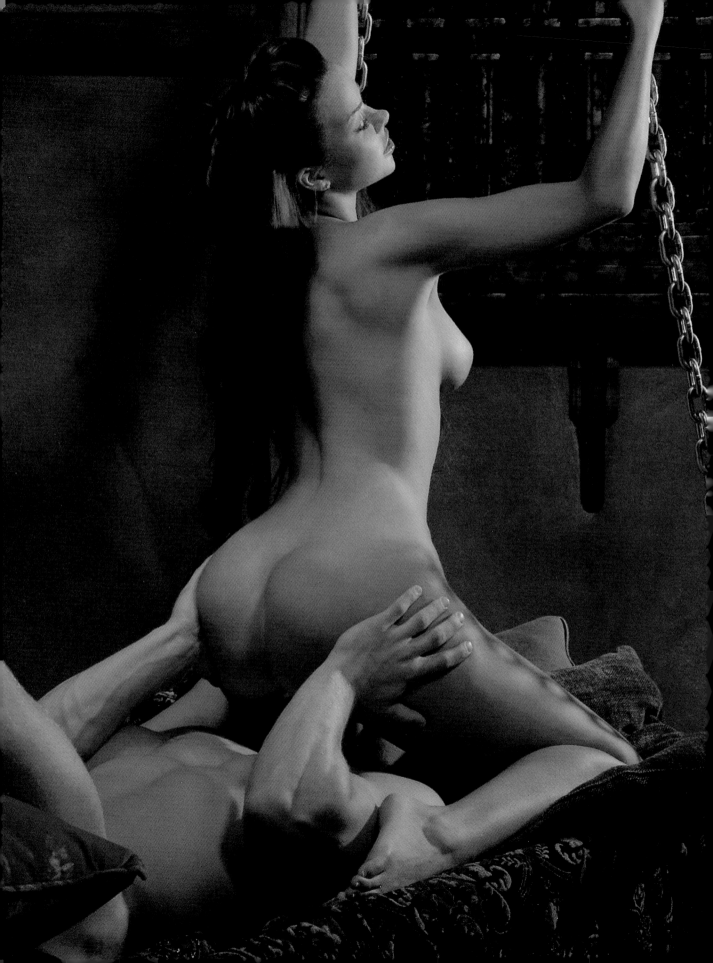

12

Art
Supplies:

*Resources for
Going Down*

TOYS

Babeland
7007 Melrose Avenue
Los Angeles, CA 90038
323-634-9480
www.babeland.com

DevineToys
1919B West Clay Street
Houston, TX 77019
646-229-6462
www.devinetoys.com

Freddy and Eddy
12613 Venice Boulevard
Los Angeles, CA 90066
310-915-0380
www.freddyandeddy.com

Good Vibrations
1620 Polk Street (at Sacramento Street)
San Francisco, CA 94109
415-345-0400
www.goodvibrations.com

JT's Stockroom
2807 West Sunset Boulevard
Los Angeles, CA 90026
1-800-755-TOYS
www.stockroom.com

Sliquid Lubricants
6046 Penrose Avenue
Dallas, TX 75206
1-800-Sliquid
www.sliquid.com

WEBSITES

AfroErotik (www.afroerotik.com)
An amazing collection of African-American themed erotica.

All About the Penis (www.allaboutthepenis.com)
The title says it all, but the tone is irreverent and fun.

Clitical (www.clitical.com)
Got clitoris questions? Clitical has the answers.

Embody Tantra (www.embodytantra.com)
A wealth of information on all things Tantric from the mind and heart of Deva Charu, Tantric Mistress.

Freddy and Eddy (www.freddyandeddy.com)
Our own website devoted to sexuality for all couples.

Hidden Self (www.hiddenself.com)
Jenn Ramsey's personal website devoted to her never-ending search for giving and receiving the ultimate oral orgasm.

Sex Info 101 (www.sexinfo101.com)
More than oral sex, this site includes almost all topics sexual and has a nifty positions guide.

Sexuality.org (www.sexuality.org)
An amazing compendium of sexual information on oral sex, massage, and everything in-between.

Sliptongue (www.sliptongue.com)
Hot erotic stories to heat you up before the pants come down.

Tiny Nibbles (www.tinynibbles.com)
Oral orator Violet Blue's site covers your adventures going down from head to toe.

Wild in Secret (www.wildinsecret.com)
Online retailer of sexual products known for their terrific service and support.

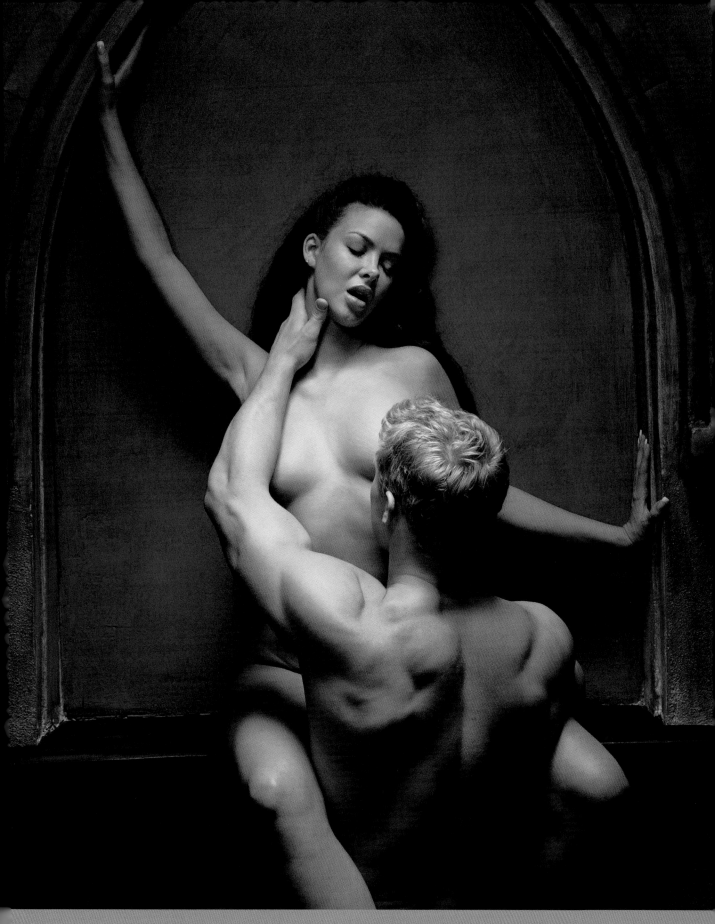

DVDS

Better Oral Sex Techniques. Dr. Marty Klein, Sinclair Intimacy Institute (1997).

Freddy and Eddy's Guide to Going Down. Alexander Institute (2007).

Modern Tantra Workshop. Dr. Patti Britton, Alexander Institute (2006).

Nina Hartley's Advanced Guide to Oral Sex. Adam and Eve Productions (2006).

Tantric Massage for Lovers. Steve Carter, Institute for Ecstatic Living (2005).

BOOKS

Blackledge, Catherine. *The Story of V.* Piscataway, NJ: Rutgers University Press (2004 edition).

Block, Joel D. *The Art of the Quickie.* Beverly, MA: Quiver Books (2006).

Blue, Violet. *The Ultimate Guide to Cunnilingus: How to Go Down on a Woman and Give Her Exquisite Pleasure.* San Francisco, CA: Cleis Press (2005 edition).

Blue, Violet. *The Ultimate Guide to Fellatio: How to Go Down on a Man and Give Him Mind-Blowing Pleasure.* San Francisco, CA: Cleis Press (2005 edition).

Cadell, Ava. *The Pocket Idiot's Guide to Oral Sex.* New York, NY: Alpha Books (2006 edition).

Chia, Mantak and Maneewan; Abrams, Douglas; and Carlton, Rachel. *The Multi-Orgasmic Couple: Sexual Secrets Every Couple Should Know.* New York, NY: HarperCollins (2002).

Chia, Mantak and Maneewan. *The Multi-Orgasmic Man: Sexual Secrets Every Man Should Know.* New York, NY: HarperCollins (1997).

Franklin, Jacqueline. *The Ultimate Kiss: Oral Lovemaking, A Sensual Guide for Couples.* Los Angeles: Media Press (2001 edition).

Hite, Shere. *The Hite Report: A Nationwide Study of Female Sexuality.* New York, NY: Seven Stories Press (2004 edition).

Kinsey, Alfred Charles. *Sexual Behavior in the Human Male.* Philadelphia, PA: W.B. Saunders and Co. (1948 edition).

O'Hara, Kristen. *Sex as Nature Intended It.* Hudson, MA: Turning Point Publications (2002 edition).

Reich, Wilhelm. *The Function of Orgasm: Discovery of the Orgone.* New York, NY: Farrar, Straus and Giroux (1986).

Zopol, Felicia. *Let's Talk About Sex: More Than 600 Quotes on the World's Oldest Obsession.* Philadelphia, PA: Running Press Publishers (2002).

ACKNOWLEDGMENTS

We'd like to acknowledge Deva Charu Morgan for her tantric wisdom, guidance, and contribution to this book. Special thanks to Jason and Angela Leach, Bob Nelson, Scottie Lowe, Dr. Patti Britton, Dr. Marty Klein, Kim Airs, Jamye Waxman, Jordan Dawes, Jordan Paul, Jenn Ramsey, Paul Sanchez, Jane Dalea-Kahn, Jagatjoti, Dean Elliott, Rachel Venning, Larry Chizek, Nina Helms, Robert Berryman, Audacia Ray, Juli Crockett, Scott and Melody, Trina Lance, Robert Scott Leyse, Steven and Amanda, Al Vitaro, and Violet Blue for your constant support and sex positive attitudes in helping make the world a better place.

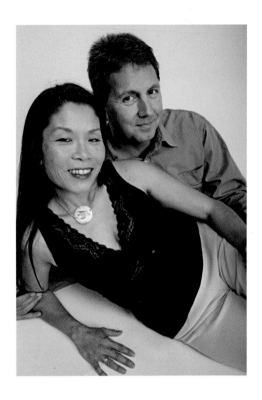

ABOUT THE AUTHORS

In 2001, husband and wife team Ian and Alicia Denchasy left their careers in teaching and law, respectively, in search of deeper sexual connection within the context of their marriage. Today, they operate www.freddyandeddy.com, a hugely popular destination site for couples interested in enhancing their sex lives.

    The duo, who have been together for almost eighteen years, also write a weekly column—read by over 1.3 million people—in both the *LA Weekly* and the *Orange County Weekly*. They live in a house with a white picket fence with their son in Los Angeles, California.